Study Guide

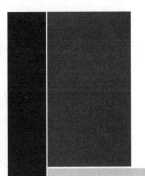

Introduction to Clinical Pharmacology

Fifth Edition

Marilyn Winterton Edmunds, PhD, ANP/GNP
Adjunct Faculty
Johns Hopkins University
School of Nursing
Baltimore, Maryland

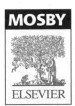
MOSBY
ELSEVIER

W9-AEZ-026

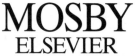

11830 Westline Industrial Drive
St. Louis, Missouri 63146

STUDY GUIDE
INTRODUCTION TO CLINICAL PHARMACOLOGY, Fifth Edition

ISBN 13   9780323032230
ISBN 10   0323032230

NOTICE

Knowledge and best practice in this field are constantly changing. As new research and experience broaden our knowledge, changes in practice, treatment and drug therapy may become necessary or appropriate. Readers are advised to check the most current information provided (i) on procedures featured or (ii) by the manufacturer of each product to be administered, to verify the recommended dose or formula, the method and duration of administration, and contraindications. It is the responsibility of the practitioner, relying on their own experience and knowledge of the patient, to make diagnoses, to determine dosages and the best treatment for each individual patient, and to take all appropriate safety precautions. To the fullest extent of the law, neither the Publisher nor the Author assumes any liability for any injury and/or damage to persons or property arising out or related to any use of the material contained in this book.

The Publisher

ISBN 13   9780323032230
ISBN 10   0323032230

NCLEX®, NCLEX-RN®, and NCLEX-PN® are federally registered trademarks and service marks of the National Council of State Boards of Nursing, Inc.

Executive Publisher: Barbara Nelson Cullen
Acquisitions Editor: Lee Henderson
Associate Developmental Editors: Laura Chu, Catherine Ott
Publishing Services Manager: Deborah L. Vogel
Senior Project Manager: Deon Lee

The author wishes to thank Joyce LeFever Kee and Evelyn R. Hayes for permission to reuse drug labels from their book, *Pharmacology, A Nursing Process Approach,* 4th edition.

Printed in the United States of America

Last digit is the print number: 9 8 7 6 5 4 3 2 1

Contents

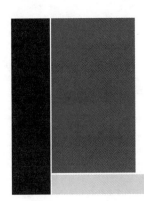

To the Student

This study guide was created to assist you in achieving the objectives of each chapter in *Introduction to Clinical Pharmacology*, and establishing a solid base of knowledge in pharmacology. Completing the exercises in each chapter in this guide will help to reinforce the material studied in the textbook and learned in class. Such reinforcement also helps students to be successful on the NCLEX-PN®.

STUDY HINTS FOR ALL STUDENTS

Ask Questions!

There are no stupid questions. If you do not know something or are not sure, you need to find out. Other people may be wondering the same thing but may be too shy to ask. The answer could mean life or death to your patient. That is certainly more important than feeling embarrassed about asking a question.

Chapter Objectives

At the beginning of each chapter in the textbook are objectives that you should have mastered when you finish studying that chapter. Write these objectives in your notebook, leaving a blank space after each. Fill in the answers as you find them while reading the chapter. Review to make sure your answers are correct and complete. Use these answers when you study for tests. This should also be done for separate course objectives that your instructor has listed in your class syllabus.

Key Terms

At the beginning of each chapter in the textbook are key terms that you will encounter as you read the chapter. Text page number references are provided for easy reference and review, and the key terms are in color the first time they appear in the chapter. Phonetic pronunciations are provided for terms that students might find difficult to pronounce. The terms that were assigned simple phonetic pronunciations were selected because they are either (1) difficult medical, nursing, or scientific terms or (2) other words that may be difficult for students to pronounce. The goal is to help the student reader with limited proficiency in English to develop a greater command of the pronunciation of scientific and nonscientific English terminology. It is hoped that a more general competency in the understanding and use of medical and scientific language may result.

Key Points

Use the Key Points at the end of each chapter in the textbook to help with review for exams.

Reading Hints

When reading each chapter in the textbook, look at the subject headings to learn what each section is about. Read first for the general meaning. Then reread parts you did not understand. It may help to read those parts aloud. Carefully read the information given in each table and study each figure and its caption.

Concepts

While studying, put difficult concepts into your own words to see if you understand them. Check this understanding with another student or the instructor. Write these in your notebook.

Class Notes

When taking lecture notes in class, leave a large margin on the left side of each notebook page and write only on right-hand pages, leaving all left-hand pages blank. Look over your lecture notes soon after each class, while your memory is fresh. Fill in missing words, complete sentences and ideas, and underline key phrases, definitions, and concepts. At the top of each page, write the topic of that page. In the left margin, write the key word for that part of your notes. On the opposite left-hand page, write a summary or outline that combines material from both the textbook and the lecture. These can be your study notes for review.

Study Groups

Form a study group with some other students so you can help one another. Practice speaking and reading aloud. Ask questions about material you are not sure about. Work together to find answers.

References for Improving Study Skills

Good study skills are essential for achieving your goals in nursing. Time management, efficient use of study time, and a consistent approach to studying are all beneficial. There are various study methods for reading a textbook and for taking class notes. Some methods that have proven helpful can be found in *Saunders Student Nurse Planner: A Guide to Success in Nursing School*. This book contains helpful information on test-taking and preparing for clinical experiences. It includes an example of a "time map" for planning study time and a blank form that you can use to formulate a personal time map.

ADDITIONAL STUDY HINTS FOR ENGLISH AS SECOND-LANGUAGE (ESL) STUDENTS

Vocabulary

If you find a nontechnical word you do not know (e.g., *drowsy*), try to guess its meaning from the sentence (e.g., *With electrolyte imbalance, the patient may feel fatigued and drowsy*). If you are not sure of the meaning, or if it seems particularly important, look it up in the dictionary.

Vocabulary Notebook

Keep a small alphabetized notebook or address book in your pocket or purse. Write down new nontechnical words you read or hear along with their meanings and pronunciations. Write each word under its initial letter so you can find it easily, as in a dictionary. For words you do not know or for words that have a different meaning in nursing, write down how they are used and sound. Look up their meanings in a dictionary or ask your instructor or first-language buddy. Then write the different meanings or usages that you have found in your book, including the nursing meaning. Continue to add new words as you discover them. For example,

primary
- of most importance; main: *the primary problem or disease*
- the first one; elementary: *primary school*

secondary
- of less importance; resulting from another problem or disease: *a secondary symptom*
- the second one: *secondary school (in the United States, high school)*

First-Language Buddy

ESL students should find a first-language buddy—another student who is a native speaker of English and who is willing to answer questions about word meanings, pronunciations, and culture. Maybe your buddy would like to learn about your language and culture. This could help in his or her nursing experience as well.

The Nursing Process

Answer Key: A complete answer key was provided for your instructor.

OBJECTIVES

1. List the five steps of the nursing process.
2. Discuss how the nursing process is used in administering medications.
3. Identify subjective and objective data.
4. List specific nursing activities related to assessing, diagnosing, planning, implementing, and evaluating the patient's response to medications.

⊕ **Be sure to check out the bonus material on the free CD-ROM in your textbook, including:**

Audio Pronunciation Guide
NCLEX®-Style Review Questions: Chapter 1
Video Clips
- Right Medication
- Right Time
- Right Dose
- Right Patient
- Right Route
- Documentation

WORKSHEET 1-1   Subjective and Objective Information

For each item listed, indicate whether it is a subjective or an objective finding by placing an "**S**" or an "**O**" in the space provided. Assume that the patient is hospitalized and some information is already known.

1. _____ Patient's age
2. _____ Complaint of pain
3. _____ Excessive gas and bloating
4. _____ Dizziness
5. _____ Pulse rate
6. _____ Dyspnea
7. _____ Pallor
8. _____ Rales in the lungs
9. _____ Wheezing
10. _____ Shortness of breath
11. _____ Vomiting
12. _____ Nausea
13. _____ Cramps in the legs
14. _____ Weight gain
15. _____ Cough
16. _____ Bruising
17. _____ Headache
18. _____ Tenderness
19. _____ Elevated blood pressure
20. _____ Blood glucose level

WORKSHEET 1-2   Components of the Nursing Process

For each of the items listed below, indicate what part of the nursing process describes this nursing activity. Place an "**A**" for assessment, "**D**" for diagnosis, "**P**" for planning, "**I**" for implementation, or "**E**" for evaluation in the space provided. Some items may be important in more than one part of the nursing process.

1. _____   Chief complaint of the patient

2. _____   Duration of drug action

3. _____   Peptic ulcer

4. _____   Action of the drug

5. _____   Family history of illness and disease

6. _____   Dosage of the medication

7. _____   History of allergy

8. _____   Severe nausea caused by radiation therapy

9. _____   Blood pressure

10. _____   Site of last injection

11. _____   Electrocardiogram

12. _____   Time last pain medication was given

13. _____   Side or adverse effects of the drug

14. _____   Special precautions in giving medication

15. _____   Expected action of the drug

16. _____   Contraindications to administration of drug

17. _____   Z-track injection technique

18. _____   Acute myocardial infarction

WORKSHEET 1-3   Nursing Drug History

Mr. Tracy Jones, a tall, thin, 67-year-old African American man, is brought to the hospital unit from the emergency room. Mr. Jones was released from this hospital 1 month ago following a myocardial infarction (heart attack). He returns today complaining of severe chest pain. His wife reminds you that he also has diabetes and high blood pressure.

Use the information presented in this case to answer the following questions.

1. What statements can you make about the patient's need for medication?

2. What are two other important areas you need to explore in completing the drug history for this patient?

    a.

    b.

3. There are different kinds of information a nurse may use in collecting the history. A primary source is the patient. The nurse may also rely on previous records or laboratory findings. These are authoritative sources of information about the patient and his health. The patient's condition may make it necessary for the nurse to ask questions of other individuals. This is secondary information about what people have observed. Finally, information may be collected from general sources that might provide information about a particular problem. Give an example of specific information you might learn from primary, secondary, and tertiary sources that might provide important information in assessing Mr. Jones' medication needs.

    a. Information from primary source

    b. Information from secondary source

    c. Information from tertiary source

WORKSHEET 1-4   Planning Drug Therapy

Mr. Jones is having a great deal of chest pain. The doctor has ordered "Nitroglycerin 0.4 mg SL tablet stat and repeat in 3 minutes if the pain is not gone."

Read about nitroglycerin in your text (see index).

1. When nitroglycerin is ordered, what is the therapeutic goal for Mr. Jones?

2. What important information needs to be known about this drug before it is given?

3. Are there special storage precautions? Administration procedures? Techniques for administration? Equipment needs?

    Describe.

4. What would you want to teach Mr. Jones about this medicine?

WORKSHEET 1-5   The Drug Order

The drug order is written on the order sheet as directed by institutional policy. The order sheet should have the patient's name and room number stamped on each sheet. The order must be signed by a licensed prescriber to be valid and should be written legibly so there is no question as to meaning. Each drug order should contain the following information.

1. The date medication was ordered

2. The name of the medication

3. The dosage of the medication

4. The time the medication is to be given

5. The route of administration

6. How many doses are to be administered

7. Any special instructions

Example of a typical drug order

_____

_____

_____

_____

_____

_____

_____

_____

_____

_____

_____

_____

_____

_____

2 Patient Teaching and Health Literacy

Answer Key: A complete answer key was provided for your instructor.

OBJECTIVES

1. List some of the problems that patients have when they cannot read or understand health instructions.
2. Identify the common causes of patient medication errors.
3. Describe the process of teaching patients about medications.

Be sure to check out the bonus material on the free CD-ROM in your textbook, including:

Audio Pronunciation Guide
NCLEX®-Style Review Questions: Chapter 2
Animations
- Patient Noncompliance

WORKSHEET 2-1   Helping Patients Become Compliant

There are two basic reasons why patients have difficulty following their treatment plans: they do not understand what they should do, or they understand what they should do but fail to do it. They may not believe that they need to carry out the treatment plan. If they do believe they should do something, they may fail to carry out the plan because they might not have the money, time, or ability to do it. The nurse, in teaching the patient, must have the ability to discuss both reasons and help patients meet their treatment goals.

1. What do you believe is the problem in the following case?

    You go out to lunch with your friend who has just been diagnosed with diabetes. She orders a fresh fruit salad, a caffeinated soda, and has a slice of zucchini bread. She tells you she can't have sugar in her coffee any more.

    What would you do?

2. Your teenage daughter is in college. She says that she can't afford to buy fruits or vegetables because they cost so much money. She knows she should eat better, but has to make choices about how she spends her money and would rather eat pizza.

    What would you do?

3. Mrs. Maxwell is prescribed digitalis in the morning, a beta blocker twice a day, a diuretic three times a day, ASA 82 mg every day, and calcium 1200 mg every evening. You notice that she has lots of medicine left over from the last time she filled her prescription, so you know she isn't taking her medicine as ordered.

    How would you handle this?

WORKSHEET 2-2   Communicating with the Patient (Health Literacy)

1. Identify some of the things that make it difficult for you and the patient to talk to each other.

2. What are some of the things that make health-related materials difficult for patients to understand?

3. If you were to prepare some educational handouts for patients, what would be some of the things you might consider?

4. How could you write or explain the following paragraphs more simply?

    a. When you arise, take your antiinfectives prior to eating your breakfast.

    b. One of the potential complications of the medicine is nephrotoxicity.

    c. Drug interactions may cause adverse reactions.

    d. Notify your health care professional if you have any hematological symptoms.

WORKSHEET 2-3   The Process of Patient Education

Deciding what the patient needs to know

1. How would you find out what the patient wants to know?

2. How would you teach the patient who doesn't want to know the things you want to teach him?

3. What are the benefits and problems in using the following teaching methods?

Teaching Method	Benefits	Problems
Verbal instructions		
Written materials		
Audiovisual materials		
Demonstrations		
Combinations of these methods		

4. How can you tell if the patient has learned what you are trying to teaching him?

5. What are some helpful teaching tips in working with patients?

6. What should you remember about reading level in creating patient teaching materials?

7. List some ideas that would be helpful as you write your own materials or select published handouts that you might want to use for your patients. Keep in mind that the goals of the material should be stated clearly.

8. Using these ideas, prepare information that encourages patients to wash their hands before handling their medications.

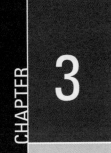

CHAPTER 3

Legal Aspects Affecting the Administration of Medications

Answer Key: A complete answer key was provided for your instructor.

OBJECTIVES

1. List the names of major federal laws about drugs and drug use.
2. Explain what is meant by "scheduled drugs" or "controlled substances" and give examples of drugs in the different schedules.
3. List rules of states and agencies that affect how nurses give drugs.
4. Explain how the nurse is responsible for controlled substances.
5. List what information is included in a medication order or prescription.
6. Define and give examples of the four different types of medication orders.
7. Describe the differences between authority, responsibility, and accountability.
8. List what you need to do if you make a medication error.

◉ **Be sure to check out the bonus material on the free CD-ROM in your textbook, including:**

Audio Pronunciation Guide
NCLEX®-Style Review Questions: Chapter 3

WORKSHEET 3-1   Classifying Drugs

Using your text, look up the following medications and, based on the information provided, try to classify each medication according to whether you believe it might be a **"CS"** for controlled substance, **"PD"** for prescription drug, or may be purchased **"OTC"** for over-the-counter.

Note: Some medications may have more than one classification, based on dosage.

1. _____   Diazepam
2. _____   Phenobarbital
3. _____   Mylanta
4. _____   Ampicillin
5. _____   Ortho-Novum
6. _____   Benadryl
7. _____   Metamucil
8. _____   Ceclor
9. _____   Tussi-Organidin
10. _____   Colace
11. _____   Robitussin-AC
12. _____   Theo-Dur
13. _____   Ibuprofen

WORKSHEET 3-2   Identifying Parts of the Patient's Chart

Traditional sections of the patient's chart include the following.

a. Summary sheet
b. Graphic record
c. History and physical examination
d. Problem list

e. Progress notes
f. Laboratory tests
g. Consultations
h. Physician's orders

Indicate in which part or parts of the patient's chart you would look for the following information.

1. _____   Blood pressure

2. _____   Report from the cardiologist

3. _____   Bed rest with bathroom privileges

4. _____   Major diagnosis

5. _____   Weight

6. _____   Description of heart sounds

7. _____   Tetracycline 500 mg PO four times daily

8. _____   Barium enema on Thursday

9. _____   Enema given

10. _____   Response to pain medication

11. _____   Intake and output record

12. _____   Electrolyte report

13. _____   CBC with differential on Thursday

14. _____   Occupation

15. _____   Insurance

WORKSHEET 3-3   More Practice Understanding Medication Orders

Explain the following drug orders. Classify the order as an **"SO"** for standing order, **"Stat"** for stat order, **"PRN"** for prn order, or **"S"** for single order.

Classification   **Explanation of drug order**

1. _____   Demerol 100 mg IM stat _____

2. _____   MOM 30 mL PO hs _____

3. _____   Seconal 100 mg PO hs prn _____

4. _____   Lanoxin 0.25 mg PO qd _____

5. _____   Dilantin 100 mg PO _____

6. _____   Monistat vaginal suppositories I q hs x 10 days _____

7. _____   Metamucil l T in glass cold water q AM ac _____

8. _____   Proventil inhaler ii puffs orally prn wheezing _____

9. _____   Lo/Ovral 1 qd PO x 21 days _____

10. _____   Entex LA ½ tab q12h prn congestion _____

11. _____   ASA gr x PO _____

12. _____   Tigan 200 mg suppository PR q6h if nauseated _____

WORKSHEET 3-4   Legal Aspects Surrounding the Administration of Medications

. The head nurse, Mrs. Jones, is getting ready to leave the hospital unit after a 12-hour shift. Mrs. Brown is the nurse just coming on duty. The two nurses meet at the locked narcotic box to complete the inventory count required at the end of each shift. During the count, it is discovered that 1 100 mg ampule of Demerol is missing. Discuss the following strategies that should be taken to solve this discrepancy and determine why you would do each of these things.
   a. Check with other nurses.
   b. Check charts of patients receiving Demerol.
   c. Check charts of patients going to surgery.
   d. If medication cannot be accounted for, notify nursing supervisor, nursing office, or hospital security.

Multiple Choice

. One of the doctors asks you if he can borrow the key to the narcotics box because he needs to give a patient some medicine before she leaves for a procedure. You should
   1. give him the key but make sure he signs out the narcotic on the sign-out sheet.
   2. open the narcotics box for him and give him the medicine, but do not give him the key.
   3. call the nursing supervisor because the doctor should never be given narcotics.
   4. tell the doctor that if he will write the order, you will be happy to give the patient the narcotic.

. What is the difference between controlled substances and prescription drugs?
   1. All drugs sold in drug stores are controlled over-the-counter drugs.
   2. The Food and Drug Administration considers all medications to be controlled substances.
   3. Controlled substances have a greater potential for abuse.
   4. Controlled substances are not available through prescriptions.

. A wide variety of medications are available over the counter. Patients often do not report to their health care provider that they are taking these products. Why might this be a problem?
   1. Because they could become addicted to the over-the-counter product.
   2. Because some over-the-counter products may interact adversely with prescription drugs that may be ordered.
   3. Because the patient taking two different types of drugs could then become dependent on the prescription drugs.
   4. It would not be a problem because over-the-counter products are of a very low dosage.

. Miss Lawson was hurrying to give the patient her medication and did not read the medication card carefully. She gave the patient 2500 mg tetracycline instead of 250 mg. She should
   1. tell the patient immediately what has happened.
   2. discuss the problem with the head nurse and physician to determine what to do.
   3. note the error in the patient chart and fill out an accident report. (Because this is an antibiotic, there is no risk of overdosage.)
   4. Check the patient's vital signs to make certain he or she is still breathing.

WORKSHEET 3-5   Ethical Situations to Ponder

1. You see a coworker secretly slip some medications into her pocket.

2. You have been at work for 5 hours and have a terrible headache. Two hours ago, you took some ibuprofen you brought from home and it did not help. There are some drug samples of new medications in the cabinet. Should you take something for your headache?

3. You are the nurse passing medications on your team. The nurses' station is very busy and there are lots of new admissions. It is 2 PM and you realize that you forgot to pass the 1 PM medications.

4. The patient is disoriented and restless. When you approach her to give her the medication cup, she knocks the pills on the floor. The next delivery from the pharmacy will not be on your shift.

5. The doctor orders two very expensive antibiotics from the pharmacy. When you mix them together in the IV fluid, a thick white cloud forms in one layer of the IV fluid.

4 Foundations and Principles of Pharmacology

nswer Key: A complete answer key was provided for your instructor.

BJECTIVES

. Define the key words used in pharmacology and about giving drugs.
. Explain the differences between the chemical, generic, official, and brand names of medicines.
. Describe the four basic physiologic processes that affect medications in the body.
. List the basic types of drug actions.
. Discuss the differences between side effects and adverse effects.

Be sure to check out the bonus material on the free CD-ROM in your textbook, including:

Audio Pronunciation Guide
NCLEX®-Style Review Questions: Chapter 4
Animations
- Receptor Interaction
- Agonists/Antagonists
- Comparison of Drug Absorption by Route of Administration
- Bioavailability of Oral Drugs
- Passive Diffusion
- Drug Movement Through the Body
- Distribution: Fat- vs. Water-Soluble Drugs
- The Effect of Protein Binding When the Volume of Distribution is Large
- The Effect of Protein Binding When the Volume of Distribution is Small
- Phase I and Phase II Biotransformation Reactions
- Sites of Drug Metabolism: First-Pass Metabolism in the Liver
- Cytochrome P-450 Drug Metabolism
- Enzyme Induction—Examples of CYP Inducers
- Enzyme Inhibition—Examples of CYP Inhibitors
- Drug-Drug Interaction: Displacement of Drug from Binding Proteins When the V_d is Low
- Effect of Food on Drug Absorption: Gastric Emptying with Digoxin
- Effect of Drugs on Nutrient Absorption

WORKSHEET 4-1   Pharmacologic Definitions and Drug Names

1. Pharmacology is _____

2. Medicines represent _____

3. *Drugs* comes from a term meaning _____

4. Therapeutic regimen includes which of the following items?
   1. Maalox 30 cc qh
   2. Keep arm wrapped in Ace bandage
   3. Patient's weight
   4. Clear liquid diet
   5. Rales in the lungs
   6. Refer patient to Alcoholics Anonymous meeting

5. Using your text, *Mosby's GenRx*, or the *Physicians' Desk Reference*, and the *Hospital Formulary*, look up the following drugs and give their official, generic, trade, and chemical names.

	Official	Generic	Trade	Chemical
a. Aspirin				
b. Chlorothiazide				
c. Diazepam				
d. Ethacrynic acid				
e. Prednisone				

6. Look in the index of your text. Find several trade or brand names that you think were selected by the manufacturer to help physicians to remember and prescribe this drug.

WORKSHEET 4-2   Identifying Drug Processes

Absorption

. Define the term *absorption*.

. How is absorption different from adsorption?

. List three factors that influence rate of absorption.

. Classify the following drugs as fast or slow in absorption by the body:

    a. _____   Proventil bronchodilator aerosol

    b. _____   Adrenalin in oil SQ

    c. _____   Nitroglycerin SL

    d. _____   Compazine rectal suppository

    e. _____   Enteric-coated aspirin

    f. _____   Aqueous adrenalin subQ

    g. _____   Nitroglycerin patch

    h. _____   Metamucil 1 glass

Distribution

. Give two examples of factors that influence distribution.

    a.

    b.

Metabolism

. Define the term *biotransformation*.

. What is the main organ of metabolism?

Excretion

. Name two major routes of drug excretion.

. What is meant by *half-life*?

WORKSHEET 4-3   Classifying Types of Drug Reactions

Ms. Carmen, a 48-year-old patient, was admitted to the hospital with pneumonia. She has an elevated temperature, chills, and a cough that has produced a large amount of green-colored sputum. She also reports that she is severely congested and has a sore throat.

Ms. Carmen has had high blood pressure for several years and takes propranolol daily to reduce it. The patient was started on therapy consisting of 500 mg Pen-Vee K PO q6h, ASA gr x prn temperature elevation, and Robitussin cough syrup, 30 cc q4h prn.

What types of drug reactions might be experienced with the drugs she is taking?

	ASA	**Pen-Vee K**
Expected effect	_____	_____
Side effect	_____	_____
Adverse reaction	_____	_____
Allergic reaction	_____	_____

Can you anticipate any drug interactions for Ms. Carmen?

	Guaifenesin (Robitussin)	**Propranolol (Inderal)**
Expected effect	_____	_____
Side effect	_____	_____
Adverse reaction	_____	_____
Allergic reaction	_____	_____

Can you anticipate any drug interactions for Ms. Carmen?

WORKSHEET 4-4   Recognizing Types of Drug Interactions

Look up the following medications in your text to determine known drug interactions.

1.   Coumadin

2.   Ortho-Novum 1/35

3.   ASA

4.   Dilantin

5.   Flagyl

Lifespan and Cultural Modifications

Answer Key: A complete answer key was provided for your instructor.

OBJECTIVES

1. Identify specific considerations in giving medications to pediatric, pregnant, breastfeeding, or elderly patients.
2. Identify special considerations that should be taken in providing care to individuals from different cultures.
3. Describe specific nursing behaviors that assist in helping patients succeed with their medication plans.

● **Be sure to check out the bonus material on the free CD-ROM in your textbook, including:**

Audio Pronunciation Guide
NCLEX®-Style Review Questions: Chapter 5

WORKSHEET 5-1   Special Considerations in the Pediatric, Geriatric, and Pregnant or Breastfeeding Patient

1. For the purposes of giving medications, does it matter how *child* is defined?

2. The dosage requirements for young children are not always smaller than for older children. Why?

3. What special physiologic changes in adolescents affect their medications?

4. When a drug label reads "safety and efficacy for use in children not established," what does this mean?

5. In the small community in which you live, you have become very familiar with one patient over the years. He has diabetes, hypertension, and arthritis and takes many medications. What physiologic changes in his body might affect the medications he now takes compared to when you first met him?

6. Two 65-year-old men taking the same antihypertensive medication come into the clinic. One of them is very overweight and in poor physical condition, and the other patient is a very large man who plays tennis and swims every day. What one factor places the overweight individual at higher risk for drug toxicities than the patient in good physical condition?

7. An elderly patient is diagnosed with diabetes and started on insulin therapy. She has very poor vision and her hands are swollen with arthritis, making self-administration of insulin difficult. Identify some strategies, appropriate to your community, that might be helpful in solving this problem.

(Continued)

WORKSHEET 5-1	Special Considerations in the Pediatric, Geriatric, and Pregnant or Breastfeeding Patient *(cont'd)*

8. Mrs. Liddle lives alone in a retirement community. She is on a fixed income and has a hard time purchasing her medications. You discover that many of the residents of the retirement community share medications in order to reduce medical and pharmacy costs. How would you deal with this problem?

9. Leslie Kline discovers that she is pregnant. She is very upset because she has been taking an antibiotic for the last 2 weeks for a severe case of bronchitis. What would you tell her?

10. Where could you go to find out what medications Leslie could take while she is pregnant or breastfeeding?

11. Look through the text to discover some of the major drugs that are teratogens.

12. When is the riskiest time during pregnancy to take a teratogenic drug?

13. Joy Hansen has been taking anticonvulsant medication for years. She recently discovered she is pregnant. She knows many anticonvulsant drugs are teratogenic but is afraid to go off her medication. What does "weighing the benefits against the risks" mean?

14. Missy Rockwood has a 3-week-old baby. She has developed severe mastitis, and the doctor started her on a course of antibiotics for treatment. What should she do about her breastfeeding?

WORKSHEET 5-2   Products Used Throughout the Life Span

Use your text, other readings, and class discussions to fill in the following chart.

Medications	Goals of Therapy	Why
Immunizations	Children (be specific) Adults (be specific)	
Antidiabetic agents		
Hormone replacement therapy		
Cholesterol-lowering agents		
Smoking cessation		
Obesity drugs		
Contraception		
Antidepressants		
Drugs for impotence		
Aspirin		

WORKSHEET 5-3   Cultural Influences Related to Medications

1. Give examples of some apparent cultural differences that may affect health care.

2. Why do you think that health and religion might be intertwined in culture?

3. How would you find out about the beliefs of a patient from another culture?

4. In teaching a patient about his thyroid replacement medication it becomes clear that the patient feels very uncomfortable about taking medicine. How would you deal with this?

5. You see a 7-year-old child at school who has long black bruises down his back. He has missed a lot of school recently because of illness. You know that his parents are from Cambodia, that they are struggling financially, and that they are part of a strong Cambodian community. The father has been drinking heavily, and you wonder if he is abusing the child. How could you find out about the bruises?

6. You have worked with several patients from Nigeria, but you know that you don't understand some of their cultural beliefs. You ask one of your African-American colleagues for information. What message does this send?

7. When you enter the hospital room of a dying Native American you find the patient's family has thrown dirt all over him. How will you handle this situation?

8. Mrs. Chen's husband has been very ill. When she visits him in the hospital she is concerned that he is not getting better. You find that she has brought him some herbal tea to help him to "raise the hot element" in his body and "achieve balance." You do not know what is in the tea. What would you do?

WORKSHEET 5-4   Strategies to Increase Patient Success with Drug Treatment

1. What is drug noncompliance?

2. What are some of the consequences of drug noncompliance?

3. Describe a situation in which you have been noncompliant with a medication. Why?

4. In the following situations, identify the factors underlying drug noncompliance.

Situation in which drug noncompliance occurs	Factor underlying noncompliant behavior
a. Little child spits out medication	_____
b. Woman fails to take her calcium replacement	_____
c. Patient forgets daily dose of thyroid supplement	_____
d. Patient forgets to take antihypertensive medication 4 times a day	_____
e. Patient uses less nicotine replacement gum than ordered	_____
f. Nitroglycerine was outdated and carried loosely with other cardiac medications in a box	_____
g. Patient has diarrhea from medication	_____

5. What strategies would be useful to you if someone were trying to help you understand how to take your medicine?

◆ Chapter 5—Integrated Case Study ◆

As a public health nurse, you are sent to the home of Mr. Shen, an elderly Chinese man who has tuberculosis. He lives in an extended family situation in a small apartment in the inner city. Several of his family members have developed positive PPD reactions since his diagnosis and are to take prophylactic INH medications. Your community has developed many drug-resistant strains of TB and you are concerned about Mr. Shen's response to treatment. You have worked primarily with Hispanic and African American patients and know nothing about Mr. Shen's culture.

Questions to discuss as a group:

1. Discuss some of the things you need to learn about this patient and his culture.

2. How would you find out some of this information?

3. How does his living in a family rather than alone affect the care you may plan for him?

4. If this man or his family does not take their medication because of cultural beliefs, it is a problem for the entire community. Explain this statement.

5. How could you obtain compliance?

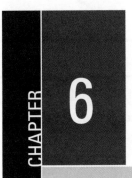

Self-Care: Over-the-Counter Products, Herbal Therapies, and Drugs for Health Promotion

Answer Key: A complete answer key was provided for your instructor.

OBJECTIVES

1. List advantages and disadvantages of over-the-counter medications.
2. Describe some of the precautions to think about in taking herbals or other alternative or complementary therapies.
3. Identify common agents taken for health promotion.

Be sure to check out the bonus material on the free CD-ROM in your textbook, including:

Audio Pronunciation Guide
NCLEX®-Style Review Questions: Chapter 6

WORKSHEET 6-1   Over-the-Counter Drug Usage

1. Identify a variety of sources that patients may have for information about over-the-counter drug use.

2. How many of these sources might provide high-quality information for patients?

3. Many patients believe that if a medication is available without a prescription, it must be safe. In what situations might OTC products pose a risk to patients?

4. Name some OTC products that might be particularly harmful to pediatric or geriatric patients.

5. New federal requirements have been passed for OTC package labeling. How could patients make certain they were using an OTC product appropriately and safely?

6. How might you discover the extent to which your patient is using OTC therapy?

7. Think about each of the key items essential to explain to patients about OTC use. Be prepared to explain why each item is important. How are these items important in children?

WORKSHEET 6-2   Alternative or Complementary Therapies and Nutritional Supplements

1. What is the difference between alternative and complementary therapy?

2. When might complementary therapy be appropriate?

3. What are the risks of alternative therapy?

4. Where can you obtain reliable information about herbal and complementary therapy?

5. Safety, purity, and effectiveness are the major issues in evaluating herbal products. Important questions to consider in evaluating herbal products for therapy include

    a.

    b.

    c.

    d.

    e.

(Continued)

WORKSHEET 6-2   Alternative or Complementary Therapies and Nutritional Supplements *(cont'd)*

6. What is aromatherapy and when might it be used?

7. When might vitamins or minerals be prescribed as a therapeutic regimen?

8. What is a free radical and how does it develop?

9. How do antioxidants help to reduce the incidence of atherosclerosis or cancer?

10. What are natural sources of antioxidants?

◆ Chapter 6—Integrated Case Study ◆

Jeannie Boyer and her husband are excited about having a baby. They talk to the nurse midwife about what they can do before conception to help ensure that they have a healthy baby. The nurse midwife recommends taking folic acid. Jeannie doesn't want to do this because she is afraid any medication might hurt the fetus when she gets pregnant. She has always been told by her mother never to take any medicine when she is pregnant.

1.   What would you tell Jeannie about folic acid and the risk to the fetus?

Because of your education, Jeannie changes her mind and goes to the pharmacy to buy the folic acid. She finds several other vitamin and mineral preparations that claim to be beneficial for her and the baby. She buys several different multivitamins and takes 3 to 4 times the recommended dosage. She feels that "more would be better" where vitamins are concerned.

2.   What would you tell her about the large dosage of vitamins?

3.   Jeannie gets pregnant but continues to work in a very stressful job. Are there any alternative therapies that might help her deal with the additional fatigue she feels?

After the baby is born, Jeannie reads about some herbal products that provide contraception. Because they are available in the natural foods store, she feels she doesn't need to visit the midwife or get a prescription.

4.   Are there any precautions you would give Jeannie?

(Continued)

◆ Chapter 6—Integrated Case Study *(cont'd)* ◆

Several months after the baby is born, Jeannie develops thrombophlebitis and is in acute pain. She has read that acupuncture would be a good treatment for this problem.

5.   Do you agree? Why or why not?

6.   If you don't know whether this is a good treatment, how would you find out?

Review of Mathematical Principles

Answer Key: A complete answer key was provided for your instructor.

OBJECTIVES

1. Work basic multiplication and division problems.
2. Interpret Roman numerals correctly.
3. Apply basic rules in calculations using fractions, decimal fractions, percentages, ratios, and proportions.

Be sure to check out the bonus material on the free CD-ROM in your textbook, including:

Audio Pronunciation Guide
NCLEX®-Style Review Questions: Chapter 7
Drug Calculator

REVIEW SHEET
MULTIPLICATION FACTS

Reprinted from the text is the basic number grid for multiplication. Find the two numbers you wish to multiply. Draw a line from one number on the left side of the chart and one line down from the other number in the top column. The answer is where the two lines intersect. Any number times zero is zero. Any number times one is itself.

MULTIPLICATION AND DIVISION GRID

	2	3	4	5	6	7	8	9	10	11	12
2	4	6	8	10	12	14	16	18	20	22	24
3	6	9	12	15	18	21	24	27	30	33	36
4	8	12	16	20	24	28	32	36	40	44	48
5	10	15	20	25	30	35	40	45	50	55	60
6	12	18	24	30	36	42	48	54	60	66	72
7	14	21	28	35	42	49	56	63	70	77	84
8	16	24	32	40	48	56	64	72	80	88	96
9	18	27	36	45	54	63	72	81	90	99	108
10	20	30	40	50	60	70	80	90	100	110	120
11	22	33	44	55	66	77	88	99	110	121	132
12	24	36	48	60	72	84	96	108	120	132	144

Now calculate the following multiplication problems. Do not use the grid unless you must.

Symbols for multiplication include x, •, or ( ).

1. 9 x 5 =

2. (8) (7) =

3. 7 • 6 =

4. (11) (4) =

5. 9 • 3 =

WORKSHEET 7-1   Reviewing Multiplication Facts

1.
$$\begin{array}{r} 23 \\ \times\ 15 \\ \hline \end{array}$$

2.
$$\begin{array}{r} 213 \\ \times\ 19 \\ \hline \end{array}$$

3.
$$\begin{array}{r} 321 \\ \times\ 11 \\ \hline \end{array}$$

4.
$$\begin{array}{r} 179 \\ \times\ 16 \\ \hline \end{array}$$

5. $200 \times 15 =$

6. $387 \times 35 =$

7. $789 \times 106 =$

8. $2305 \times 3211 =$

9. $21 \times 19 =$

10. $(34)\ (59) =$

11. $843 \times 79 =$

12. $1798 \times 0 =$

13. $436 \times 212 =$

14. $(79)\ (64) =$

15. $341 \times 26 =$

16. $2002 \cdot 1007 =$

17. $329{,}472 \times 3 =$

18. $(246)\ (835) =$

19. $(404)\ (103) =$

20. $(601)\ (47) =$

21. $(333)\ (58) =$

22. $201 \cdot 34 =$

23. $7530 \cdot 341 =$

24. $47{,}347 \cdot 6 =$

25. $3400 \times 21 =$

26. $198 \times 4 \times 1 =$

27. $163 \times 3 \times 7 =$

REVIEW SHEET
DIVISION FACTS

Divide when you see the symbol ÷ (as 12 ÷ 4 =); the symbol — (as $\frac{12}{4}$); the symbol / (as 12/4); or the symbol $\lceil$ (as $4 \lceil 12$).

Each of these would be read as 12 divided by 4.

In the problem $4 \lceil \overset{3}{12}$:

The number being divided (12 in the problem above) is called the *dividend*.

The number doing the dividing (4 above) is called the *divisor*.

The number in the answer (3 above) is called the *quotient*.

If the number cannot be divided into equal groups the number left is the *remainder*. If the remainder is more than half the divisor, round the quotient up 1 number. If it is less than one half, leave the quotient as it is.

For example:

$$
\begin{array}{r}
24 \\
25\,\overline{\smash{)}\,600} \\
\underline{50} \\
100 \\
\underline{100}
\end{array}
\qquad
\begin{array}{r}
24 \\
25\,\overline{\smash{)}\,603} \\
\underline{50} \\
103 \\
\underline{100} \\
3\ r
\end{array}
\qquad
\begin{array}{r}
24 \\
25\,\overline{\smash{)}\,624} \\
\underline{50} \\
124 \\
\underline{100} \\
24\ r
\end{array}
$$

Therefore, the third quotient will be rounded up to 25.

Look back to the grid reprinted from the text for basic multiplication facts. This grid can also be used for division. On the left side of the chart, find the number you are dividing with. Look across the column for the number you wish to divide. If the number is there, look up the column to find the number that is the exact quotient of the two numbers. If the number is not there, find the closest number. If the number in the chart is slightly larger than the one you want, you will have a remainder. If the number in the chart is slightly smaller, you will have to use a number one less in the quotient. For example, 6 into 42 is exactly 7, while 8 into 50 is 6 with a 2 remainder. Dividing 6 into 29 yields 4 with a 5 remainder.

WORKSHEET 7-2   Reviewing Division Facts

Now calculate the following division problems. Do not use the grid unless you must.

1. $3 \overline{)213}$

2. $2 \overline{)2,010}$

3. $3 \overline{)70,896}$

4. $4 \overline{)2080}$

5. $5 \overline{)196,420}$

6. $7 \overline{)12,607}$

7. $2880 \div 45 =$

8. $4992 \div 39 =$

9. $8024 \div 136 =$

10. $3 \overline{)9034}$

11. $11 \overline{)123}$

12. $142 \div 12 =$

13. $25 \overline{)25,026}$

14. $17 \overline{)3416}$

15. $3429 \div 17 =$

16. $29 \overline{)10,859}$

17. $50 \overline{)1019}$

18. $428 \overline{)10,843}$

19. $100 \overline{)1027}$

20. $200,305 \div 2 =$

REVIEW SHEET
ROMAN NUMERALS

Roman numerals and their values

I = 1	C = 100
V = 5	D = 500
X = 10	M = 1000
L = 50	

Rules in using Roman numerals

1. Whenever a Roman numeral is repeated, or when a smaller numeral follows a larger one, the values are added together. For example:

    II = 2 (1 + 1 = 2)
    LVII = 57 (50 + 5 +1 + 1 = 57)
    CXIII = 113 (100 + 10 + 1 + 1 + 1 = 113)

2. Whenever a smaller Roman numeral comes before a larger Roman numeral, subtract the smaller value. For example:

    IV = 4 (5 – 1 = 4)
    CD = 400 (500 – 100 = 400)

3. Numerals are never repeated more than three times in a sequence. For example:

    III = 3
    IV = 4

4. Whenever a smaller Roman numeral comes between two larger Roman numerals subtract the smaller number from the numeral following it. For example:

    XIX = 19 (10 + [10 – 1] = 19)
    XCIX = 99 ([100 – 10] + [10 – 1] = 99)

In expressing dosages in the apothecaries' system, lower case rather than capital Roman numerals are used. A dot is always placed over the Roman numeral I whenever lower case numbers are used. For example, iii or vi is the proper form in this system rather than III or VI.

WORKSHEET 7-3   Working with Roman Numerals

Use the information on the review sheet to change the following Roman numerals into Arabic, and the Arabic numerals to Roman numerals.

1.   11 =

2.   16 =

3.   63 =

4.   77 =

5.   9 =

6.   XLIV =

7.   XXXII =

8.   XV =

9.   CDIV =

10. XXVI =

11. 6 =

12. 44 =

13. 49 =

14. 400 =

15. 83 =

16. 40 =

17. XIV =

18. LXII =

19. XCIX =

20. XXX =

21. LXXV =

22. XIV =

REVIEW SHEET
FRACTIONS

A fraction is one or more equal parts of a unit. It is written as two numbers separated by a line, such as 1/2 or 3/4. The parts of the fraction are called the *terms*. The two terms of a fraction are the **numerator** and the **denominator**. The numerator is the top number; the denominator is the bottom number.

<u>1</u> = numerator   <u>3</u> = numerator
2 = denominator   4 = denominator

The denominator tells into how many equal parts the whole has been divided. The numerator tells how many of the parts are being used.

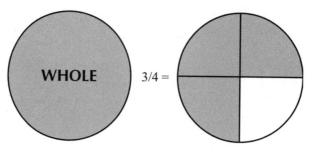

It is important to not confuse these two parts of the fraction. One way to help you remember which part belongs where is to think of the word nude. The NUmerator is on top; the DEnominator is on the bottom.

$$\frac{\begin{array}{c}N\\U\end{array}}{\begin{array}{c}D\\E\end{array}}$$

Fractions may be *raised to higher terms* by multiplying both numerator and denominator by the same number. Fractions are *reduced to lower terms* by dividing both terms of the fraction by the same number. The value of the fraction is not changed when it is lowered or raised in terms.

For example:

To raise 3/4 to a higher term multiply both the numerator and the denominator by 2, converting it to 6/8. The two fractions, 3/4 and 6/8, have the same value.

To lower 3/9 to a lower term, divide both numerator and denominator by 3, converting it to 1/3; 3/9 and 1/3 have the same value.

Proper fractions have a numerator smaller than the denominator. The number 3/4 is a proper fraction because it represents less than 1.

Improper fractions have a numerator the same as or larger than the denominator. The number 6/4 is an improper fraction because the numerator (6) is larger than the denominator (4).

In using fractions in calculations, the numerator and the denominator must be of the same unit of measure. For example, if the numerator is in grains, the denominator must be in grains.

A *mixed number* is a whole number and a proper fraction. Examples of mixed numbers include: 4 1/3; 3 3/4; 5 16/35.

(Continued)

REVIEW SHEET
FRACTIONS *(cont'd)*

is often necessary to change an improper fraction to a mixed number or to change a mixed number to an improper frac-
on when doing certain calculations. To change an improper fraction to a mixed number, divide the denominator into the
umerator. The result (quotient) is the whole number. The remainder is placed over the denominator of the improper frac-
on.

or example: 17/3 is an improper fraction. To convert to a mixed number:

. Divide the denominator (3) into the numerator (17):

$$\begin{array}{r} 5 \qquad \text{quotient} \\ \text{divisor}\quad 3\,\overline{)\,17} \\ \underline{15} \\ 2 \qquad \text{remainder} \end{array}$$

. Move the remainder (2) over the denominator (3)

$\dfrac{2}{3}$ = remainder
= denominator

. Put the quotient (5) in front of the fraction.

5 2/3

o change a mixed number 5 2/3 to an improper fraction, multiply the denominator of the fraction (3) by the whole num-
er (5) add the numerator (2), and place the sum over the denominator. For example:

The sum (17) goes over the denominator of the fraction:
17/3 is the improper fraction.

A *complex fraction* has a fraction in either its numerator or its denominator, or both. For example:

$$\dfrac{\frac{1}{5}}{50} \quad \text{or} \quad \dfrac{30}{\frac{2}{3}} \quad \text{or} \quad \dfrac{3\frac{1}{2}}{\frac{1}{8}}$$

Complex fractions may be changed to whole numbers, proper, or improper fractions, by dividing the number or fraction
above the line by the number or fraction below the line.

For example: Change $\dfrac{\frac{1}{2}}{100}$ to a proper fraction as follows:

$$\dfrac{\frac{1}{2}}{100} = \dfrac{1}{2} \div \dfrac{100}{1} = \dfrac{1}{2} \times \dfrac{1}{100} = \dfrac{1}{200}$$

Remember: When dividing fractions, invert or put upside down the divisor and then multiply.

100/1 becomes 1/100.

WORKSHEET 7-4   Review of Basic Information on Fractions

A. Indicate whether the following are proper fractions (**PF**), improper fractions (**IF**), mixed numbers (**MN**), or complex fractions (**CF**).

1. 3/4

2. 3 2/3

3. $\dfrac{\frac{1}{5}}{50}$

4. 3/1

5. 8/7

6. $\dfrac{\frac{2}{3}}{20}$

7. 8 3/5

8. 1/8

B. Change the following improper fractions to mixed numbers.

1. 13/3

2. 25/4

3. 3/2

4. 6/5

5. 18/7

6. 46/15

7. 4/3

8. 22/3

C. Change the following mixed numbers to improper fractions.

1. 4 2/3

2. 6 1/3

3. 7 3/4

4. 5 1/12

5. 3 4/5

6. 1 7/8

7. 3 1/2

8. 6 1/2

REVIEW SHEET
ADDITION OF FRACTIONS

f fractions have the same denominator, simply add the numerators, and put the sum above the common denominator. For xample:

$$\frac{2}{12} + \frac{3}{12} + \frac{5}{12} = \frac{10}{12} \quad \frac{\text{(sum of } 2 + 3 + 5)}{\text{(same denominators)}}$$

f the fractions have different denominators, they must be converted to a number that each denominator has in common, or *common denominator*. You can always find a common denominator by multiplying the two denominators by one another. ometimes, however, both numbers will go into a smaller number. For example: $1/12 + 3/8 + 3/4 = ?$ What is the smallest ommon denominator?

.   The smallest whole number that all denominators (12, 8, and 4) have in common is 24; 24, then, is the lowest common denominator.

.   Divide the smallest common denominator by the denominator of each fraction and multiply both terms of the fraction by the quotient (divide 12, 8, and 4 into 24 and multiply the numerator and denominator by the answer). This is often easier to see if we write the problem vertically:

$$\frac{1}{12} = \frac{?}{24} \qquad 24 \div 12 = 2 \qquad \frac{1}{12} \times \frac{2}{2} = \frac{12}{24}$$

$$+ \frac{3}{8} = \frac{?}{24} \qquad 24 \div 8 = 3 \qquad \frac{3}{8} \times \frac{3}{3} = \frac{9}{24}$$

$$+ \frac{3}{4} = \frac{?}{24} \qquad 24 \div 4 = 6 \qquad \frac{3}{4} \times \frac{6}{6} = \frac{18}{24}$$

3.   Then add the numerators and bring down the denominator:

$$\frac{2}{24}$$

$$+ \frac{9}{24}$$

$$+ \frac{18}{24}$$

$$\frac{29}{24}$$

4.   Reduce the improper fraction to its lowest terms by changing the improper fraction to a mixed number.

$$29/24 = 1\ 5/24$$

5.   If you are adding mixed numbers, first change them to improper fractions and proceed as above.

WORKSHEET 7-5   Practice Adding Fractions

Add the following fractions, converting improper fractions to mixed numbers in the lowest terms.

1.   7/8 + 5/8 =

2.   3/4 + 1/6 =

3.   1/16 + 5/24 =

4.   1 5/6 + 3 5/9 =

5.   3/8 + 1/8 =

6.   3/4 + 2/4 =

7.   4 4/5 + 2/5 =

8.   1 2/7 + 3 6/7 =

9.   6 3/4 + 2 =

10. 5/9 + 7/12 =

11. 1/8 + 3/16 =

12. 1 5/9 + 2 1/3 =

13. 5 3/5 + 6 3/5 =

14. 6 7/10 + 4 1/4 =

15. 1 1/2 + 1 1/4 + 1 1/8 =

16. 1 5/6 + 3 5/9 =

17. 5 1/5 + 2 2/5 =

18. 3 2/7 + 4/7 =

19. 1 3/4 + 3 3/8 =

20. 4 5/6 + 2 1/8 =

REVIEW SHEET
SUBTRACTION OF FRACTIONS

fractions have the same denominator, subtract the smaller numerator from the larger numerator. Leave the denominators e same, and then reduce to the lowest terms, if necessary. For example:

$$\frac{5}{10} - \frac{1}{10} = \frac{4}{10} = \frac{2}{5}$$

fractions do not have the same denominator, change the fractions so they have the smallest common denominator, sub-act the numerators, and leave the denominator the same. For example:

$$\frac{15}{28}$$

$$-\frac{3}{14}$$

ince 28 is a multiple of 14 (14 x 2 = 28), 28 is a common denominator of 28 and 14. Divide the smallest common denom-ator by the denominator of each fraction and multiply the numerator and denominator of the fraction by the quotient.

$$\frac{15}{28} = \frac{15}{28} \quad \text{(no change necessary)}$$

$$-\frac{3}{14} \quad x \quad \frac{2}{2} = \frac{6}{28}$$

ubtract the numerators and leave the denominators the same.

$$\frac{15}{28} - \frac{6}{28} = \frac{9}{28}$$

f you are subtracting mixed numbers, first change them to improper fractions and proceed as above.

$$2\frac{2}{3} - 1\frac{1}{6} =$$

$$\frac{8}{3} - \frac{7}{6} =$$

$$\frac{16}{6} - \frac{7}{6} =$$

$$\frac{9}{6} = 1\frac{3}{6} = 1\frac{1}{2}$$

WORKSHEET 7-6   Practice Subtracting Fractions

1. 5/8 – 3/8 =

2. 5/6 – 7/9 =

3. 4 1/4 – 3 3/8 =

4. 7/10 – 3/10 =

5. 5/18 – 3/18 =

6. 5/6 – 1/4 =

7. 7/8 – 7/40 =

8. 3/4 – 1/2 =

9. 1/4 – 1/5 =

10. 3 – 1/4 =

11. 7 – 3/5 =

12. 5 – 1 2/3 =

13. 4 – 3 1/8 =

14. 3 1/3 – 1 2/3 =

15. 6 3/10 – 3 7/10 =

REVIEW SHEET
MULTIPLICATION OF FRACTIONS

hen multiplying fractions, reduce all terms to their smallest terms to make calculations more simple. For example, 12/24 the same as 1/2, but 12/24 is much more difficult to work with. Reducing to the lowest terms is done when you can di- de the same number into both the numerator and the denominator (i.e., 2/10 can be divided by 2, therefore 2/10 equals 5; 9/36 can be divided by 9, therefore 9/36 equals 1/4).

hen the fractions are in their simplest form, multiply the numerators together, and then multiply the denominators to- ther. For example:

$$\frac{1}{20} \quad x \quad \frac{5}{3} \quad x \quad 3 \quad =$$

Remember . . .

Because 3 is a whole number it is the same as 3/1.
The 1 can be added as a denominator if it makes it easier to understand.

---

reducing, this can be simplified as follows:

$$\frac{1}{20} \quad x \quad \frac{5}{3} \quad x \quad 3 \quad = \quad \frac{1}{4} \quad x \quad \frac{1}{3} \quad x \quad \frac{3}{1}$$

$$= \quad \frac{3}{12}$$

$$= \quad \frac{1}{4}$$

the number is a mixed number (a whole number and a fraction), change it to an improper fraction before solving. For ample:

$$2\frac{1}{2} \quad x \quad \frac{2}{3} \quad x \quad 6 \quad = \quad \frac{5}{2} \quad x \quad \frac{2}{3} \quad x \quad \frac{6}{1}$$

$$\text{Simplify:} \quad = \quad \frac{5}{1} \quad x \quad \frac{1}{1} \quad x \quad \frac{2}{1}$$

$$= \quad \frac{10}{1}$$

$$= \quad 10$$

WORKSHEET 7-7 Practice Multiplying Fractions

Make equivalent fractions.

1. 1/6 = _____ /12

2. 2/3 = _____ /15

3. 7/9 = 56/ _____

4. 1/7 = _____ /28

5. 3/9 = _____ /27

Multiply the following fractions, converting to the lowest terms, and changing improper fractions to mixed numbers.

6. 2/5 • 7/8 =

7. 1/2 • 4/3 • 1/2 =

8. 2/3 • 9/4 =

9. 2/7 • 49/4 =

10. 11/12 • 12/11 =

11. 3 • 1/9 =

12. (11/17) (34/11) (1/2) =

13. (2/5) (25/10) (3/8) =

14. (1/27) (54/2) (18/1) =

15. (9) (1/3) (3/4) (1/5) =

REVIEW SHEET
DIVISION OF FRACTIONS

To divide a fraction by a fraction, invert (or turn upside down) the divisor and then multiply.

For example:

$$\frac{4}{6} \div \frac{2}{6} = ?$$

Invert the divisor

$$\frac{4}{6} \times \frac{6}{2} = ?$$

Simplify, then multiply numerators and then denominators.

$$\frac{\cancel{4}^2}{\cancel{6}_1} \times \frac{\cancel{6}^1}{\cancel{2}_1} = ?$$

$$\frac{2}{1} \times \frac{1}{1} = \frac{2}{1} = 2$$

If the number is a mixed number, change it to an improper fraction before solving. For example:

$$\frac{2}{3} \div 1\frac{1}{3} = ?$$

Change mixed number to an improper fraction:

$$\frac{2}{3} \div \frac{4}{3} = ?$$

Invert divisor:

$$\frac{2}{3} \times \frac{3}{4} = ?$$

Simplify:

$$\frac{2^1}{\cancel{3}_1} \times \frac{\cancel{3}^1}{\cancel{4}_2} = ?$$

$$\frac{1}{1} \times \frac{1}{2} = \frac{1}{2}$$

WORKSHEET 7-8   Practice Dividing Fractions

Divide the following fractions, reducing to lowest terms.

1. $4/5 \div 3/10 =$

2. $8 \div 2/3 =$

3. $5/9 \div 3/4 =$

4. $6/7 \div 3 =$

5. $3/8 \div 6/7 =$

6. $1/6 \div 1/3 =$

7. $4/6 \div 2/3 =$

8. $5/9 \div 2/5 =$

9. $3\ 1/2 \div 2\ 2/3 =$

10. $4\ 2/3 \div 1/3 =$

11. $1\ 2/3 \div 2\ 1/2 =$

12. $6\ 1/2 \div 2 =$

13. $1\ 3/4 \div 5\ 1/4 =$

14. $3/5 \div 3/10 =$

15. $2/5 \div 5/8 =$

REVIEW SHEET
DECIMAL FRACTIONS

A decimal fraction is one whose denominator is 10 or some multiple of 10. Instead of writing the denominator, a decimal point is added to the numerator.

For example:

$$1/4 = 25/100 = 0.25$$

All numbers to the left of the decimal point represent whole numbers. Those numbers to the right represent fractions. Zeros may be placed to the right of the decimal for a whole number only, without changing the value of the whole number (i.e., 45 is the same as 45.0 or 45.00).

Decimals increase in value from right to left; they decrease in value from left to right. Decimals increase in value in multiples of 10. Each column in a decimal has its own value, according to where it lies from the decimal point (see the box below).

DECIMAL POINT

Left of decimal point	Right of decimal point
Units	Tenths
Tens	Hundredths
Hundreds	Thousandths
Thousands	Ten thousandths
Ten thousands	Hundred thousandths
Hundred thousands	Millionths

654321.123456

Addition and Subtraction of Decimal Fractions:

Place the numbers so that the decimal points fall in a straight line. Keep the columns straight. Add zeros to the right if necessary. Then add or subtract as you would for whole numbers. The decimal point goes in the answer just below the decimal points in the problem.

For example: add 0.0678 and 1.082

```
   0.0678
+  1.0820   (add one zero)
   1.1498
```

The decimal point is in line with the other decimal points. Subtract 3.053 from 6.046:

```
   6.046
-  3.053
   2.993
```

(Continued)

REVIEW SHEET
DECIMAL FRACTIONS *(cont'd)*

Multiplication and Division of Decimal Fractions:

To multiply decimal fractions, multiply the two numbers and count off from right to left as many decimal places in the product (answer) as there were in the multiplier and multiplicand. For example:

$$
\begin{array}{r}
44.61 \\
\times\ \ 2.3 \\
\hline
13383 \\
8922\ \ \\
\hline
102.603
\end{array}
$$

44.61 Multiplicand (has 2 decimal places)

x   2.3 Multiplier (has 1 decimal place)

102.603 Count off 3 places right to left and insert decimal point.

To divide by a decimal fraction, first move the decimal point in the divisor (the number you are dividing with) enough places right to make it a whole number. Then move the decimal point in the dividend (the number you are dividing) as many places as it was moved in the divisor, adding zeros if necessary. Place the decimal point in the quotient (answer) directly above that in the dividend.

For example: divide 32.80 by 8.2.

8.2 $\overline{\smash{)}\ 32.80}$ 8.2 is the divisor; 32.80 is the dividend

Move the decimal point in the divisor to the right to make it a whole number, then move it the same number of places in the dividend.

82. $\overline{\smash{)}\ 328.0}$

Solve the problem:

$$
\begin{array}{r}
4.0 \\
82.\ \overline{\smash{)}\ 328.0} \\
328.0
\end{array}
$$

Because the decimal system is built on multiples of 10, a short cut may be taken when multiplying or dividing by 10, 100, or 1000. To multiply a decimal fraction by 10, 100, or 1000, move the decimal place as many places to the right as there are zeros in the multiplier. For example:

0.0006 x 1000 = ?

In 1000 there are three zeros, so

0.0006 x 1000 = 0000.6 = 0.6

To divide a decimal fraction by 10, 100, or 1000, move the decimal place as many places to the left as there are zeros in the divisor. For example:

0.5 / 100 = ?

100 has 2 whole number zeros, so

0.5 / 100 = 0.005

WORKSHEET 7-9　　Practice with Decimal Fractions

Change the following decimals to fractions:

1. .807 =

2. .0207 =

3. .12347 =

4. .666 =

5. .01 =

6. 1.3 =

Convert to common fractions or mixed numbers in lowest terms:

7. .202 =

8. 3.14 =

9. 103.004 =

10. 0.75 =

11. 0.40 =

12. 2.125 =

13. .6 =

14. .33 =

15. .26 =

Find:

16. 7.456 + .923 + 1.04 + 7.3 =

17. 31.8579 + 11.264 + 32.79 =

18. 17.77 − 6.5 =

19. 4.03 − 2.1856 =

20. 2.231 x .32 =

21. 213 x 1.28 =

22. .172 x .012 x 12 =

23. .00572 x 100 =

24. 100 x .0453 =

25. 9.128 ÷ .028 =

REVIEW SHEET
RATIOS AND PERCENTS

Ratios

A *ratio* is a way of expressing the relationship of one number to another number or of expressing a part of a whole number. The relationship is expressed by separating the numbers with a colon (:). The colon means division. The expression 1:2 is read as there is one part to two parts. Ratios are commonly used to express concentrations of a drug in solution.

For example, a ratio written as 1:20 means 1 part to 20 parts. A ratio may also be written as a fraction (e.g., 1:10 is the same as 1/10).

Percent

The term *percent* or the symbol % means parts per hundred. Thus, the percentage may also be expressed as a fraction or as a decimal fraction. For example:

30% means 30 parts per hundred or 30/100
70% means 70 parts per hundred or 70/100

Percents should also be reduced to their lowest common denominator, when appropriate. For example:

20% is 20/100 or 1/5
40% is 40/100 or 2/5

To *change a fraction to a percent*, divide the numerator by the denominator and multiply the results (quotient) by 100 and add a percent sign (%). For example:

To change 8/10 to a percent:	To change 2/5 to a percent:
$8 \div 10 = 0.8$	$2 \div 5 = 0.4$
$0.8 \times 100 = 80\%$	$0.4 \times 100 = 40\%$

To *change a mixed number to a percent*, first change it to an improper fraction, then proceed as above. For example:

To change 1 1/3 to a percent:

$$\frac{4}{3} = 4 \div 3 = 1.33 \text{ remainder } 1$$

$1.33 \times 100 = 133 \ 1/3\%$

To *change a ratio to a percent*, the ratio is first expressed as a fraction. The first number or term of the ratio becomes the numerator and the second number or term becomes the denominator (e.g., 1:200 becomes 1/200). The fraction is then changed to a percent as shown above.

1:200 = 1/200
$1 \div 200 = 0.005$
$0.005 \times 100 = 0.5\%$

To *change a percent to a ratio*, the percent becomes the numerator and is placed over the denominator of 100.

For example, to change 20% and 50% to ratios:

20% is 20/100 = 1/5 or 1:5
50% is 50/100 = 1/2 or 1:2

(Continued)

A percent may easily be expressed as a decimal, a fraction or as a ratio.

Example: 20% = 0.20 = 20/100 = 1/5 = 1:5

It is very easy to change between decimals, fractions, percents, and ratios. The following rules are presented to summarize these changes:

Rules for Changing Between Percents, Decimals, Fractions, and Ratios

To *change a fraction to a ratio*, write the two numbers with a colon between them instead of the dividing line.

Example: 1/5 = 1:5

To *change a fraction to a decimal fraction*, divide the numerator by the denominator.

Example: 1/5 = 0.20

To *change a fraction to a percent*, divide the numerator by the denominator (use as many decimal places as needed); then move the decimal point two places to the right and add the percent sign.

Example: 1/5 = 0.20 = 20%

To *change a percent to a decimal fraction*, move the decimal point two places to the left and omit the percent sign.

Example: 10% = 0.10

To *change a percent to a fraction*, drop the percent sign, write the number as the numerator, with 100 as the denominator, and reduce to the lowest terms.

Example: 10% = 10/100 = 1/10

To *change a percent to a ratio*, drop the percent sign, use the number as the first term, 100 as the second term, and reduce to the lowest terms; or change to a fraction and then use a colon instead of the dividing line.

Example: 10% = 10/100 = 1/10 or 1:10
10% = 1/10 = 1:10

To *change a decimal fraction to a percent*, move the decimal point two places to the right (multiply by 100) and add the percent sign.

Example: 0.20 = 20%

To *change a decimal fraction to a common fraction*, omit the decimal point and place the number over the appropriate denominator of 10, 100, or 1000, and reduce to the lowest terms.

Example: 0.20 = 20/100 = 1/5

To *change a decimal fraction to a ratio*, write the number as the first term; then put 10, 100, or 1,000 as the second term; finally, reduce to the lowest terms.

Example: 0.20 = 20:100 or 1:5

To *change a ratio to a fraction*, write the numbers with a dividing line instead of a colon.

Example: 1:20 = 1/20

To *change a ratio to a decimal fraction*, divide the first term by the second term.

Example: 1:20 = 0.05

To *change a ratio to a percent*, divide the first term by the second term, move the decimal point two places to the right in the answer, and add a percent sign.

Example: 1:20 = 0.05 = 5%

WORKSHEET 7-10   Practice with Ratios and Percents

Change to percents.

1. .32 =   2.   2 1/6 =   3.   2/5 =

Change to decimal fractions.

4.   67% =   5.   105% =   6.   1/4% =

7.   Change 14 2/7% to a common fraction in its lowest terms:

8.   Express 233 1/3% as a mixed number:

9.   Write 4 1/5 as a decimal:

10. Write 48% as a decimal:

11. Write 15% as a fraction reduced to its lowest terms:

12. Write 1.79 as a percent:

13. Write 1.25 as a percent:

14. Write 2 1/4 as a percent:

Ratios:

15. Write a ratio that expresses 10,000 people to a mile:

16. Ratio of 1 stamp for every dollar of purchase:

17. 7 to 4:

18. 2 eggs to 1 person:

19. 1/2 to 1/3:

20. 24 cans to 2 cases:

21. 2 feet to 7 feet:

22. 12 to 1:

23. 1 1/2 to 1 3/4:

24. 1000 square miles per person:

25. 3000 raindrops per yard:

REVIEW SHEET
PROPORTIONS

A proportion is a way of expressing a relationship of equality between two ratios. In other words, the first ratio listed is equal to the second ratio listed. The two ratios are separated by a double colon (::), which means, "as." The numbers of each end of the relationship are the extremes, and the two numbers in the middle are the means. *The product of the extremes equals the product of the means.* This means that if one of the terms is not known, it may be calculated. The unknown term is defined by an x. For example:

$$5{:}500 \ {::} \ 2{:}x$$

(when x is the unknown) means

"The relationship of 5 to 500 is the same as the relationship of 2 to x."

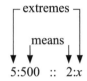

5 and x are the extremes; 500 and 2 are the means.

Proportions may be written as fractions. To find x, express the proportion as a relationship, and solve:

$$5/500 = 2/x$$

$$2 \times 500 = 1000$$
$$5x = 1000$$
$$x = 1000/5$$
$$x = 200$$

In addition to being equal, proportions must also be written in the same system in both ratios (e.g., minims is to grains as minims is to grains; ml is to grams as ml is to grams). For example:

15m: 60gr :: 13m: $x$gr   Correctly written

15m: 60m :: 13m: $x$gr   Incorrectly written

The calculation of ratios provides one of the major foundations in drug dosage calculation. Often the nurse knows the desired concentration of a drug and needs to calculate how much to give of a medication on hand. The nurse can figure how much medication to give by using the principles of proportion.

WORKSHEET 7-11   Practice with Proportions

Calculate the following, rounding decimals to the nearest hundredth:

1. $\dfrac{3.6}{2.9} = \dfrac{x}{4.3}$

2. $\dfrac{6.15}{12} = \dfrac{17.39}{x}$

3. $\dfrac{19.056}{x} = \dfrac{3.72}{16.57}$

4. $\dfrac{5}{6} = \dfrac{x}{42}$

5. $\dfrac{3}{4} = \dfrac{9}{x}$

6. $\dfrac{x}{8} = \dfrac{12}{48}$

7. $\dfrac{7}{x} = \dfrac{8}{120}$

8. $\dfrac{1\frac{1}{2}}{\frac{1}{2}} = \dfrac{x}{4}$

9. $\dfrac{\frac{2}{3}}{\frac{10}{15}} = \dfrac{4}{x}$

10. $\dfrac{x}{1\frac{1}{5}} = \dfrac{\frac{35}{42}}{\frac{4}{3}}$

11. $\dfrac{\frac{5}{9}}{x} = \dfrac{\frac{3}{4}}{1\frac{28}{35}}$

12. $0.2:1 :: 0.6:x$

13. $\dfrac{\frac{1}{48}}{\frac{1}{32}} \times 1 =$

14. $\dfrac{0.0002}{1} \times 2000 =$

15. $10:2 :: 80:x$

Mathematical Equivalents Used in Pharmacology

Answer Key: A complete answer key was provided for your instructor.

OBJECTIVES

1. Use the apothecaries' system to convert from one measure to another.
2. Use the metric system to convert from one measure to another.
3. State the values of common household measures and their equivalents.
4. Compare the units used in the apothecaries', metric, and household measures systems.
5. Use common abbreviations and symbols to interpret and solve medication problems.

⊙ **Be sure to check out the bonus material on the free CD-ROM in your textbook, including:**

Audio Pronunciation Guide
NCLEX®-Style Review Questions: Chapter 8
Drug Calculator

REVIEW SHEET
COMMON MEASURES

Common Measurements of the Apothecaries' System

Liquid Measures
60 minims (m) = 1 fluid dram (ℨ)
8 fluid drams = 1 fluid ounce (fl oz or ℥)
16 fl ounces = 1 pint (pt or O)
2 pints = 1 quart (qt)
4 quarts = 1 gallon (gal)
480 minims = 1 ounce (oz)

Solid Measures
60 grains = 1 dram (ℨ)
8 drams = 1 ounce (oz or ℥)
480 grains = 1 ounce (oz)
12 ounces = 1 pound (lb)

Common Measurements in the Metric System

Measures of Length (meter)
1 meter (m) = 100 centimeters (cm)
1 centimeter (cm) = 0.01 meter (m)

Measures of Volume (liter)
1 decaliter (d) = 10 liters (L)
1 liter (L) = 1000 milliliters (mL) or 1000 cubic centimeters (cc)

Measures of Weight (gram)
1 kilogram (kg) = 1000 grams (gm)
1 gram (gm) = 1000 milligrams (mg)
1 milligram (mg) = 1000 micrograms (µg)

> **Key Point:** Cubic centimeters, milliliters, and grams are approximately equivalent; 1cc or 1 ml weighs approximately 1 gm.

1 cc = 1 ml = 1 gm, whereas 1 kg = 2.2 lb

Relying on what you know about the decimal system, you can change measures within the same system:

To change milligrams to micrograms:
Move decimal point three places to right.   000.00007 = 000000.07

To change micrograms to milligrams:
Move decimal point three places to left.   000000.07 = 000.00007

To change grams to milligrams:
Move decimal point three places to the right (multiply by 1000).   1.000.067 = 1000.067

To change milligrams to grams:
Move decimal point three places to the left (divide by 1000).   1345.0789 = 1.3450789

> **Key Point:** Prefixes of the metric system indicate the multiples or fractions of the unit:
>
> milli = one-thousandth   deca = ten
> centi = one-hundredth   hecto = hundred
> deci = one-tenth   kilo = thousand

WORKSHEET 8-1   Apothecaries' System

1. Change 6 pounds to apothecary ounces.

2. Change 5 quarts to pints.

3. Change 6 gallons to quarts.

4. Change 3 quarts to ounces.

5. Change 3 gallons to fluid ounces.

6. Change 12 oz to grains.

7. _____ drams = gr ix

8. gr xx = _____ drams

9. ___ oz = 1 lb

10. 120 grains = _____ drams

11. _____ minims = gr xv

12. _____ drams = m xxx

13. ss oz = gr _____

Give abbreviations for the following units.

14. cubic centimeter _____   15. ounce _____

16. minim _____   17. grain _____

18. kilogram _____   19. gram _____

20. dram _____   21. milligram _____

22. microgram _____

23. List the four common units of the apothecaries' system.

WORKSHEET 8-2   Metric System

Calculate the answers to these problems using the metric system.

1.   Change 3.4 meters to centimeters.

2.   Change 5 meters to centimeters.

3.   Change 4 meters to millimeters.

4.   5 gm = _____ mg

5.   2000 cc = _____ L

6.   1000 mL = _____ L

7.   1 mL = _____ cc

8.   100 mg = _____ gm

9.   1 mg = _____ micrograms

10. 5 gm = _____ mg

11. 1200 mg = _____ gm

12. 1.5 L = _____ mL

13. _____ L = 3000 mL

14. _____ L = 250 mL

15. 0.04 gm = _____ mg

16. _____ gm = 1.4 kg

17. 150 mg = _____ gm

18. 1 kg = _____ gm

19. 1 microgram = _____ mg

20. _____ cm = 0.02 meters

21. _____ m = 1000 cm

22. 10 L = _____ decaliter

REVIEW SHEET
COMMON MEASURES

Equivalents in the Apothecaries' and Metric Systems*

Apothecaries' System		Metric System
1 gallon (gal)	=	4000 cc or 4000 ml or 4 liters
1 qt or 32 oz	=	1000 cc or 1000 ml or 1 liter
1 pt or 16 oz	=	500 cc or 500 ml or 500 gm
1 oz or 8 drams	=	30-32 cc or 30-32 ml or 30-32 gm
1 dram, 60-64 grains, or 60-64 minims	=	4-5 cc or 4-5 ml or 4-5 gm
15-16 grains, or 15-16 minims	=	1 cc or 1 ml or 1 gm
2.2 lb	=	1000 gm or 1 kg
1 grain	=	60 or 64 mg or 0.06 gm
1/60 grain	=	1 mg

---

*   To aid in teaching the conversion processes, some approximations have been made in these equivalencies. In addition, 15 rather than 16 grains are often used in calculations; 60 is often used in place of 64. These approximations account for the variance seen in the table.

Rules for Converting from One System to Another

Units to Change	Method
Grains to grams	Divide by 15 or 16.
Grains to milligrams	Multiply by 60 or 64.
Grams to grains	Multiply by 15 or 16.
Grams to milligrams	Move decimal point three places to the right.
Milligrams to grains	Divide by 60 or 64.
Milligrams to grams	Move decimal point three places to left.
Milliliters to minims	Multiply by 15 or 16.
Minims to cc	Divide by 15 or 16.

REVIEW SHEET
HOUSEHOLD MEASURES AND THEIR EQUIVALENTS

Household Measures

60 drops (gtt)	=	1 teaspoonful (t or tsp)
3-4 teaspoonsful	=	1 tablespoonful (T or Tbsp)
2 tablespoonsful	=	1 ounce (oz)
6-8 teaspoonsful	=	1 ounce (oz)
6 ounces	=	1 teacupful
8 ounces	=	1 glass or cup

Household measures may be converted to either the apothecaries' system or to the metric system. The drop is the unit in the household system equivalent to the minim and the grain.

Conversions Between Household, Apothecaries', and Metric Systems

Household Measure	Apothecaries' System	Metric System
1 teaspoonful	1 dram or 60 minims	4 or 5 ml
1 tablespoonful	3 or 4 drams	15 or 16 ml
2 tablespoonsful	8 drams or 1 ounce	30 or 32 ml
1 teacupful	6 ounces	180 ml
1 glassful	8 ounces	240 ml

The key relationship to understand in converting household measures to other systems is that 1 drop equals 1 minim and weighs 1 grain.

WORKSHEET 8-3   Converting Between Apothecaries' and Metric Systems

Calculate the answers to these problems.

1. 0.1 mg = _____ gm

2. 15 mg = gr _____

3. 60 mg = _____ gm

4. 1 gm = gr _____

5. _____ mg = gr 1/150

6. 0.016 gm = gr _____

7. 60 mg = gr _____

8. gr 1/2 = _____ gm

9. gr 1/100 = _____ mg

10. gr viiss = _____ gm

11. gr 1/6 = _____ mg

12. 0.1 gm = _____ mg

13. 0.01 gm = _____ gr

14. 0.5 gm = _____ gr = _____ mg

15. 2.5 kg = _____ lb = _____ gm

16. 100 mg = gr _____

17. gr 1/16 = _____ gm

18. gr 1/4 = _____ gm = _____ mg

19. gr 1/150 = _____ mg

20. 0.008 gm = gr _____

WORKSHEET 8-4   Using the Household System

Calculate these problems using the household system.

1. 1 T = _____ oz = _____ dram = _____ mL

2. 1 glassful = _____ mL = _____ oz

3. 3 t = _____ gtts

4. 8 t = _____ T

5. 18 oz = _____ teacupfuls

6. 32 t = _____ oz

7. 240 gtts = _____T

8. 16 oz = _____ glassfuls

Calculate these problems converting to household, metric, or apothecaries' system.

9. 1 t = _____ drams

10. 2 t = _____ minims

11. 1 glassful = _____ oz

12. _____ kg = 2.2 lb

13. 4 t = _____ T = _____ drams

14. 8 drams = _____ oz = _____ mL

15. 16 mL= _____ T

16. 36 drams = _____ oz

17. 180 minims = _____ mL

18. m xxx = _____ drams

19. 1 t = _____ drams = _____ mL = _____ oz

REVIEW SHEET
CONVERTING TEMPERATURE READINGS BETWEEN
CENTIGRADE (CELSIUS) AND FAHRENHEIT SCALES

The key relationships to understand are:

One degree on the Fahrenheit scale equals 9/5 of one degree on the Celsius scale.
One degree on the Celsius scale equals 5/9 of one degree on the Fahrenheit scale.

The formula for converting Fahrenheit to Celsius is: $(°F - 32) \times 5/9 = °C$

For example,

Change 98° F to degrees Celsius:

$(°F - 32) \times 5/9 = °C$
$(98° - 32) = 66 \times 5/9 = 36.6° C$

The formula for converting Celsius to Fahrenheit is: $(°C \times 9/5) + 32 = °F$

For example,

Change 38.8° C to degrees Fahrenheit:

$(°C \times 9/5) + 32 = °F$
$(38.8° \times 9/5) + 32 = 102° C$

WORKSHEET 8-5   Using Celsius and Fahrenheit Scales

Calculate the following answers.

1.   40° C = _____ ° F

2.   99° F = _____ ° C

3.   36.6° C = _____ ° F

4.   45° C = _____ ° F

5.   104° F = _____ ° C

6.   37.5° C = _____ ° F

7.   101° F = _____ ° C

8.   30° C = _____ ° F

9.   95° F = _____ ° C

10. 113° F = _____ ° C

Calculating Drug Dosages

Answer Key: A complete answer key was provided for your instructor.

OBJECTIVES

1. Use formulas to determine the dosages of tablets, capsules, or liquids.
2. Use formulas to determine the total number of tablets or capsules or the amount of liquid to be ordered for a specified time.
3. Use information about the apothecaries', metric, and household measurement systems to accurately calculate drug dosages.
4. Calculate dosages for parenteral injections, including those for special preparations such as insulin.
5. Calculate flow rates for infusions.
6. List three different rules used to calculate medication dosages for children.

⊙ **Be sure to check out the bonus material on the free CD-ROM in your textbook, including:**

Audio Pronunciation Guide
NCLEX®-Style Review Questions: Chapter 9
Drug Calculator

REVIEW SHEET
Computing Oral Dosages Through Ratio-Proportion

The formula to calculate the number of capsules or tablets to order is a basic proportion problem (review proportions in student text, Chapter 7):

Dose ordered	::	Tablets or capsules per dose	=	Number of tablets or
Dose available		Drug form (tablets or capsules)		capsules per dose

Key Point:
1. First change dosages to the same unit of measurement
2. Reduce to simplest terms
3. Use common sense to check your answer

Remember: When parentheses are used in a math problem, it means to do all the calculations inside the parentheses first, then complete the rest of the problem.

The formula is the same for calculating liquid dosages. Only the unit of measure is different. For liquids use:

Dose desired	x	Drug form (minims, ml, dram)	=	Amount of liquid
Dose available				per dose

WORKSHEET 9-1   Practice Computing Oral Dosages

Calculate the following involving tablets, capsules, or liquids.

1. Desired: Aspirin gr x q4h
   Available: Aspirin 0.3 gm/tablet

2. Desired: Elixir phenobarbital gr ss q4h
   Available: Phenobarbital 16 mg/4ml

3. Desired: Chloral hydrate syrup gr viiss tid
   Available: Chloral hydrate syrup 10% solution

4. Desired: Methacycline 0.3 gm stat and 150 mg q6h x 7 days
   Available: Methacycline 150 mg capsules. How many capsules per stat dose?
   How many to order for stat + 7 days?

5. Desired: Elixir ferrous sulfate 600 mg tid with meals
   Available: Elixir ferrous sulfate 300 mg/10 mL

6. Desired: KCl 40 mEq qid
   Available: KCl 20 mEq/15 mL

7. Desired: Doxycycline 0.3 gm q12h x 8 days
   Available: Doxycycline 150 mg capsules
   Number of capsules per dose? Total number to be given?

8. Desired: Amoxicillin 500 mg q6h x 4 days
   Available: Amoxicillin 250 mg

9. Desired: Guanethidine 0.025 gm qd
   Available: Guanethidine 25 mg tablet

10. Desired: Theophylline elixir 100 mg bid
    Available: Theophylline elixir 0.05 gm/5 mL
    How many mL/dose? How many gm/dose?

(Continued)

WORKSHEET 9-1 Practice Computing Oral Dosages *(cont'd)*

Practice reading labels

11. Order is for diltiazem HCl 60 mg PO bid.

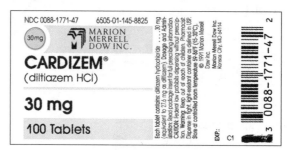

What is available? Look at the label to find this.

How much should be given?

Desired/Have =

12. Order is for Ceclor 0.5 gm PO tid.

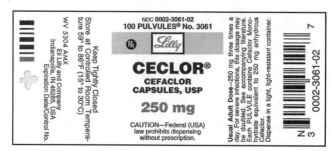

What is available? Look at the label to find this.

How much should be given?

Desired/Have =

13. Order is for Principen 200 mg PO q8h.

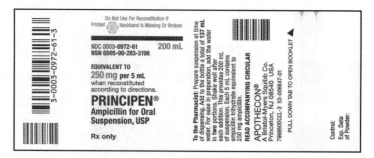

What is available? Look at the label to find this.

How much should be given?

Desired/Have =

(Continued)

WORKSHEET 9-1   Practice Computing Oral Dosages *(cont'd)*

14. Order is for digoxin 0.25 mg IM daily.

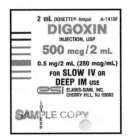

What is available? Look at the label to find this.

How much should be given?

Desired/Have =

15. Order is for heparin 4000 units subQ.

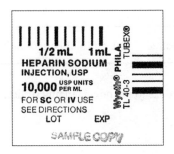

What is available? Look at the label to find this.

How much should be given?

Desired/Have =

16. Order is for hydrochlorothiazide (HydroDIURIL) 25 mg PO daily.

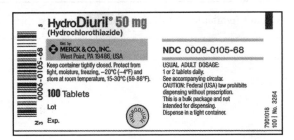

What is available? Look at the label to find this.

How much should be given?

Desired/Have =

REVIEW SHEET
COMPUTING DOSAGES OF PARENTERAL MEDICATIONS

Ratio and proportion are the standard methods of calculating parenteral dosages:

Drug Available : Dilution :: Drug Desired : x

Dose desired	x	Dilution or amount of solution	=	Amount of solution
Dose available				per dose

If instructions are not given for diluting medications, a modification of the familiar proportion formula may be used:

Dose Desired : 1 ml :: Total Drug Available : x

Note: This is not the Desired/Available formula we have been using. Desired does not always go over Available. Think about what you are looking for!

Look at the relationships in the formula:

Dose Desired : 1 ml :: Total Drug Available : x

Dose to known amount of liquid compared to dose to unknown amount of liquid.

Multiply the means, divide by the extremes.

Total drug available	x	1 ml	=	Amount of diluent required
Dose desired				to add vial powder so that
				dose ordered = 1 ml

Another time when solutions are involved is when sterile hypodermic tablets are to be administered. These special tablets are placed in a syringe and diluted, usually with 1 ml solution. The amount to be given may be computed thus:

Amount Available : 1 ml :: Amount Desired : x ml

WORKSHEET 9-2   Practice Computing Parenteral Dosages

Calculate the following problems for parenteral dosages.

1. Desired: Morphine sulfate 10 mg
    Available: Morphine sulfate 16 mg/mL

2. Desired: Penicillin G 400,000 units IM
    Available: Penicillin G 1,000,000 units/5 mL

3. Desired: Atropine sulfate gr 1/150
    Available: Atropine sulfate 0.6 mg/mL

4. Desired: Demerol 50 mg IM stat
    Available: Demerol 100 mg/2 mL

5. Desired: Tigan 200 mg IM q8h prn nausea
    Available: Tigan 0.1 gm/mL

6. Desired: Aminophylline 0.25 gm IM q4h prn wheezing
    Available: Aminophylline gr viiss/2 mL

7. Desired: Procaine penicillin G 500,000 units IM bid
    Available: Procaine penicillin G 300,000 units/mL

8. Desired: Dilaudid gr 1/32 q4h prn pain
    Available: Dilaudid 2 mg/mL

(Continued)

WORSHEET 9-2   Practice Computing Parenteral Dosages *(cont'd)*

Practice reading labels

9. Desired: Heparin 6000 units subQ

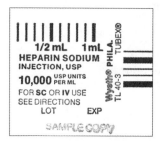

Available:

Desired/Have:

10. Desired: Kanamycin 15 mg/kg/day in three divided doses (q8h) IV. Client weighs 50 kg.
    Calculate mg desired: 15 mg/kg x 50 kg = 750 mg desired.

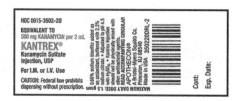

Available:

Desired/Have:

Divide into 3 equal doses =

11. Desired: Morphine sulfate gr 1/8 IM q4h prn pain.

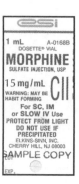

Available:

Convert to like units:

Then do ratio and proportion:

(Continued)

WORKSHEET 9-2   Practice Computing Parenteral Dosages *(cont'd)*

12. Desired: Cefamandole (Mandol) 250 mg IM q6h for a child weighing 15 kg.
    Child's recommended drug dosage is 50–100 mg/kg/day in 3 to 6 divided doses.
    Recommended dosages for this child would be:
    So recommended dosage range would be:
    Order is for 250 mg q6h so _____ is the recommended dosage range.
    Check the label to see what is available.

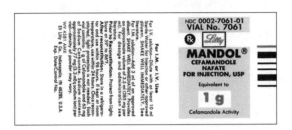

Desired: 250 mg

Available:

13. Order meperidine (Demerol) 30 mg IM stat.

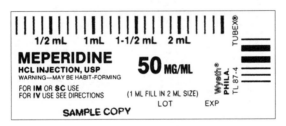

Available:

Desired/Have:

REVIEW SHEET
COMPUTING DOSAGES OF INSULIN

The calculation and preparation of insulin dosage is unique in three ways:

1. There are many different kinds of insulin, but they all come in a standardized measure called a unit. Insulin is available in 10-ml vials in two strengths: U-100 (100 units per 1 ml solution) or U-500 (500 units per 1 ml solution). As you can see, U-500 is five times stronger than U-100. (U-500 is rarely used.)

2. Insulin should be drawn up in a special insulin syringe calibrated in units. If an insulin syringe is not available, a tuberculin syringe calibrated in minims may be used.

3. The insulin order, the insulin bottle, and the insulin as drawn up should always be rechecked by another nurse for maximum accuracy. Small errors may cause big problems!

WORKSHEET 9-3   Practice Computing Insulin Dosages

State the syringe and insulin you would use and calculate the following problems for insulin:

. Order: 45 units NPH (isophane insulin suspension) U-100 1 hour before breakfast daily.

Syringe	Type Insulin	Amount
U-100	_____	_____
_____	U-500	_____

. Order: 38 units lente insulin U-100 (insulin zinc suspension) 1 hour before breakfast daily

Syringe	Type Insulin	Amount
U-100	_____	_____
TB	_____	_____

. 30 units PZI (protamine zinc insulin) U-100 and 20 units regular (Iletin) insulin U-100 30 minutes at breakfast daily.

Syringe	Type Insulin	Amount
U-100	U-100	_____
U-100	U-500	_____

. 40 units regular (Iletin) insulin U-100 30 minutes ac tid.

Syringe	Type Insulin	Amount
TB	_____	_____

. 25 units regular (crystalline zinc) insulin U-100 and NPH (isophane insulin suspension) U-100 40 units $\frac{1}{2}$ hour before breakfast daily

Syringe	Type Insulin	Amount
U-100	U-100	_____
TB	U-100	_____

(Continued)

WORKSHEET 9-3   Practice Computing Insulin Dosages *(cont'd)*

6. Read the label and answer the following questions:

   Mrs. Bennie has had an allergic reaction to NPH Iletin pork insulin. The health care provider has changed the insulin to NPH Humulin insulin 55 units subQ daily ac breakfast.

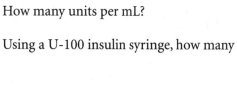

   a. What is the source of insulin?

   b. Is this the correct source of insulin?

   c. How many units per mL?

   d. Using a U-100 insulin syringe, how many units would you give?

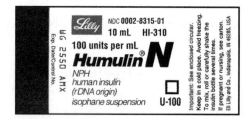

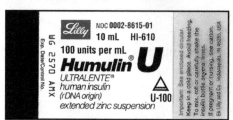

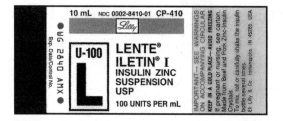

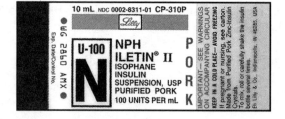

7. Order reads regular insulin 10 units and NPH insulin 25 units subQ q8AM.
   a. Study the labels above. Which of these bottles would you use to draw up regular insulin?

   b. Which of these bottles would you use to draw up NPH insulin?

   c. List in order the steps you would take to draw up the insulin.

REVIEW SHEET
CALCULATING FLOW RATES FOR INTRAVENOUS INFUSIONS

.   Calculating the flow rate for IV fluid administration.

A.   The rate at which IV fluids are given is the *flow rate* and is measured in drops per minute.
B.   *Drop factor* is the number of drops per milliliter of liquid and is determined by the size of the drops.

'he drop factor is different for different manufacturers of IV infusion equipment and must be checked by reading it on the fusion set itself. Generally, though, drop factors range between 10 and 15 drops per milliliter. Infusion sets have different rop factors for use with blood infusion sets (usually 10 to 12 drops per milliliter) because the drops are larger, while pedi-tric setups use very small drops called microdrops (often with 50 or 60 microdrops per milliliter).

> **Key Point:** The flow rate for infusions can be calculated.

> The drop factor for infusions depends upon the type of equipment and must be read from the infusion set label.

)nce the nurse has learned the drop factor for the equipment being used, the flow rate may be calculated by using the fol->wing formula:

$$\text{Drop factor} \times \text{Milliliters per minute} = \text{Flow rate (drops/min)}$$

or

$$\frac{\text{Total of fluid to give}}{\text{Total time (minutes)}} \quad \times \quad \text{Drop factor} \quad = \quad \text{Flow rate (drops/min)}$$

.   Modifying the drop rate for children.

'he drop factor must be determined from the infusion setup. Usually 60 microdrops per ml is the drop factor for infants. or calculating the flow rates in infants the same formula is used, except the microdrop drop factor must be substituted ito the formula for the adult drop factor.

$$\frac{\text{Total of fluid to give}}{\text{Total time (minutes)}} \quad \times \quad \text{Drop factor} \quad = \quad \text{Flow rate (drops/min)}$$

.   Calculating total administration time.

ometimes physicians will specify how fast they want infusions to run. The nurse needs to calculate the total time the in-
ısion will run.

'alculating total administration time for IV fluid depends on calculating the total number of drops to be infused. Using
his information, plus the drop factor, the total infusion time can easily be determined by use of the following formula:

$$\frac{\text{Total drops to be infused}}{\text{Flow rate (drops/min)} \times 60} \quad = \quad \text{Total infusion time (hr or min)}$$

WORKSHEET 9-4   Practice Computing IV Infusion Rates and Times

1. The physician orders 1000 mL 5% dextrose in water (D_5W) to be administered in 4 hours. Drop factor is 10 gtts/mL. Calculate the following.
    a. The number of minutes the medication is to flow
    b. The number of milliliters the patient will receive per minute
    c. The number of drops the patient will receive per minute

2. Give 1000 mL D_5W at 30 gtts/min. Drop factor is 15 gtts/mL. Calculate the following.
    a. The total number of drops to be given
    b. The total number of minutes to flow
    c. The total time for infusion in hours and minutes

3. Give 400 mL lactated Ringer's solution in 3 hours. The drop factor is 15 gtts/mL. Calculate the following.
    a. The total number of minutes to flow
    b. The number of mL the patient will receive per minute
    c. The number of drops per minute

4. Infuse 500 mL blood in 2 hours. Administration set has a drop factor of 10. How many drops per minute?

5. The patient was given 1000 mL normal saline in 5 hours. What was the rate of administration (flow rate) if the drop factor was 15?

6. Determine the flow rate for IV administration of 1200 mL to be given at rate of 3 mL/min. Drop factor is 15.

7. Give an infant 60 mL of IV D_5W at 0.5 mL/min. Drop factor is 60. Calculate the following.
    a. Determine the total number microdrops.
    b. Determine the total number minutes of flow.
    c. Determine the hours and minutes solution is to flow.
    d. Determine the flow rate.

8. Give an infant 90 mL IV infusion at rate of 30 microgtts/min. Drop factor is 60. Calculate the following.
    a. The total number of microdrops to be given
    b. The total number of minutes infusion is to flow
    c. The total number of hours and minutes solution is to flow

REVIEW SHEET
COMPUTING DOSAGES FOR INFANTS AND CHILDREN

Clark's rule: Based on the child's body weight.

Based on the proportion of the average adult weight and the adult dosage, we can calculate the child's dosage using the child's weight.

$$\text{Adult weight : Adult dosage :: Child's weight : } x \text{ Child's dosage}$$

Other formulas substitute kilograms for pounds in calculating the weights.

Young's rule: Used for children ages 2 to 12.

$$\frac{\text{Child's age}}{\text{Child's age} + 12} \times \text{ Adult dose } = \text{ Child's dose}$$

Fried's rule: Used for children under the age of 2.

$$\frac{\text{Infant's age in months}}{150} \times \text{ Adult dose } = \text{ Infant's dose}$$

Body surface area: Used for children when accuracy is needed. The total body surface area is determined using a nomogram or chart (see following page), and is put into the following formula:

$$\frac{\begin{array}{c}\text{Surface area of the child}\\ \text{in square meters}\end{array}}{\begin{array}{c}\text{Surface area of an adult}\\ \text{in square meters } (1.73 \text{ m}^2)\end{array}} \times \text{ Usual adult dose } = \text{ Child's dose}$$

(Continued)

REVIEW SHEET
COMPUTING DOSAGES FOR INFANTS AND CHILDREN *(cont'd)*

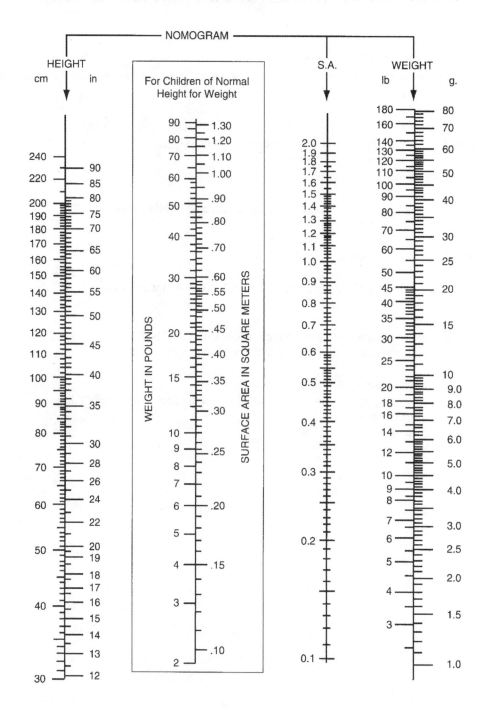

BSA nomogram. Place a straightedge from the patient's height in the left column to his weight in the right column. The point of intersection on the body surface area column indicates the body surface area (BSA).

(From Lilley LL, Harrington S, Snyder JS: *Pharmacology and the nursing process*, ed 4, St Louis, 2005, Mosby; modified from data by Boyd E, West CD, in Berhman RE, Kliegman RM, Jensen HB: *Nelson textbook of pediatrics*, ed 17, Philadelphia, 2004, WB Saunders.)

WORKSHEET 9-5   Practice Calculating Pediatric Dosages

Calculate the following dosages for children using the different rules and the nomogram for determining body surface area for children.

		Data for children			Children's dosage using			
Adult dose	Age	Weight (lb)	Height (in)		Clark	Young	Fried	BSA
1. Atropine sulfate gr 1/150	18 mo	25	32		_____	_____	_____	_____
2. Aminophylline 0.5 gm	6 yr	38	42		_____	_____	_____	_____
3. Gentamicin 80 mg	22 mo	28	33		_____	_____	_____	_____
4. Cleocin 200 mg	9 yr	52	48		_____	_____	_____	_____
5. Kantrex 0.5 gm	10 mo	22	29		_____	_____	_____	_____
6. Phenobarbital sodium gr ii	12 mo	22	31		_____	_____	_____	_____

. Compare the children's dosages among the various methods used. What are some observations you might make about the various methods? How do they compare in dosage?

(Continued)

WORKSHEET 9-5   Practice Calculating Pediatric Dosages *(cont'd)*

Practice reading labels

8. Order: Cefadroxil (Duricef) 70 mg PO q12h
    Child's weight: 20 lb
    Child's recommended drug dosage: 30 mg/kg/day
    Check the label to see what is available:

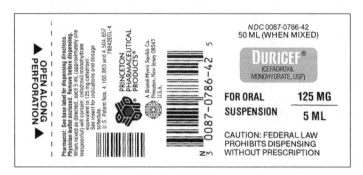

a. Available:

b. Identify the lb/kg conversion factor:

c. Use ratio and proportion to convert 20 lb to kg:

d. Calculate safe dosage range:

e. Is the prescribed drug dose within safe parameters?

f. If this dose were given, calculate dosage:

    Desired:

    Have:

g. Desired/Have =

WORKSHEET 9-6   Mastering Drug Calculations

1. The physician has ordered 0.5 gm of ampicillin IM. The label reads "1 gm ampicillin powder. For IM use, must be reconstituted with 3.5 mL of diluent. Resulting diluent contains 250 mg ampicillin per 1 mL." How much of the diluted medication do you administer to the patient?

2. The order is for digoxin (Lanoxin) 0.375 mg IV. The medication comes in 0.5 mg in 2 mL. How much of the medication should be administered? If this dose were to be given orally, would the dosage be the same?

3. Mrs. Bodkins, age 70, has type 2 diabetes and has been admitted with dehydration, confusion, vomiting, and hypotension. She has not taken her insulin and has not been eating. Her blood glucose level is 530 mg/dL. The order is to start an IV with 1000 mL of 0.45 normal saline and then give 7 units of regular insulin IV push stat and follow it with an insulin drip of 7 units per hour. The medication available is Humulin Regular 100 units per ml. If you prepared an insulin drip of 50 units of regular insulin in 50 ml of NS, how much would you infuse in 1 hour?

4. A vial of penicillin G aqueous contains 5,000,000 units (U) per vial. It may be reconstituted with different amounts of diluent to produce different concentrations according to the following.

Diluent	Concentration/mL
23 mL	200,000 U
18 mL	250,000 U
8 mL	500,000 U
3 mL	1,000,000 U

If you dilute the 5,000,000-U vial with 23 mL, how many units of penicillin are in each milliliter?

5. The pediatrician orders that an infant is to be given 350 mg Ceftin IM q6h. The medication comes in 220 mg/mL. How much should the nurse give?

REVIEW SHEET
DIMENSIONAL ANALYSIS CALCULATIONS

Anything that a nurse can do to eliminate medication errors is important. Some find that using dimensional analysis reduces frustration and confusion in dosage calculation. *Dimensional analysis* provides a single method to use for all kinds of drug problems, even those with two or three steps. This method provides a visual guide used by the nurse to construct a problem in an orderly, step-wise fashion. The numbers in the dosage calculation problem are placed on a grid along with their labels. The labels are then cross-canceled in order to assure that only one label is left – the one that is needed for the final answer. After cross-cancellation, numbers are multiplied across the top and bottom of the grid which yields a fraction. This fraction is divided and the final label applied for the answer. This method reduces the chance of incorrect placement or inversion of drug calculation factors and is especially suited for complex problems or those that call for unit conversions. An understanding of ratio and proportion provides a solid foundation for the use of dimensional analysis in dosage calculations. Following are the steps to construct a dimensional analysis problem.

The physician orders vitamin C, 1500 mg PO to be given after breakfast. Tablets on hand are 500 mg per 1 tablet (tab).

1. **Identify the final answer label.**   Look at the problem and ask, "What is the term that I will use to label the final answer to this dosage calculation?   Is it milliliters, tablets, liters?

    State, **"The final answer to this dosage calculation will be labeled as 'tablets' (tabs).**

    Ask, **"How many tablets will need to be administered to this patient?"**

    Write this question as:

    ?tab   =

2. **Draw a grid to the right of the label.**

    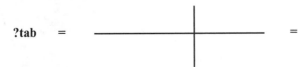

    In this format, the horizontal bar means "divide" and the vertical bar means "multiply."

3. **Find a given factor in the dosage calculation problem that is labeled with the same name as the final answer label.**

    *The physician orders vitamin C 1500 mg PO to be given after breakfast. Tablets on hand are 500 mg per **1 tablet (tab)**.*

    Insert that unit label directly to the right, and in the top or numerator position on the grid.

    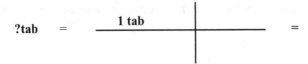

(Continued)

REVIEW SHEET
DIMENSIONAL ANALYSIS CALCULATIONS *(cont'd)*

4. **Write the numbers in the problem in the correct form that shows a relationship or ratio.**

In this case, it is given that 1 tablet contains 500 mg. of Vitamin C; in other words, 500 mg per 1 tab are available. So, with the label of 1 tab above the grid line, the corresponding term of "500 mg." is written below the line. This indicates the relationship or ratio of 1 tab to 500 mg.

$$?\text{tab} \quad = \quad \frac{1\ \text{tab}}{500\ \text{mg}} \quad \Bigg| \quad =$$

5. **Check for the given number with the same label that appears in the first, lower space or denominator position on the grid. Place the number that belongs with this label in the next upper (numerator) space of the grid.**

*The physician orders vitamin C **1500 mg** PO to be given after breakfast. On hand are 500 mg per 1 tablet (tab).*

In this problem, the given factor 1500 mg will be placed in the next grid space.

$$?\text{tab} \quad = \quad \frac{1\ \text{tab}}{500\ \text{mg}} \quad \Bigg| \quad 1500\ \text{mg} \quad =$$

6. **Cancel Labels**. After all factors in the problem have been accounted for, proceed to ***cancel out*** the unit labels by making a single diagonal line through cross-matching labels as illustrated. This is called "cross-cancellation." If the dosage calculation problem has been properly set up, only the final answer label "tab" will remain uncancelled.

$$?\text{tab} \quad = \quad \frac{1\ \text{tab}}{500\ \cancel{\text{mg}}} \quad \Bigg| \quad 1500\ \cancel{\text{mg}} \quad =$$

7. **Calculate**. All numbers above the line are multiplied horizontally, left to right. All numbers below the line are multiplied horizontally, left to right. The final answer will appear as a fraction – which is actually a division problem. Divide the top number (numerator) by the bottom number (denominator) and then attach the final answer label left (tabs) to the answer.

$$?\text{tab} \quad = \quad \frac{1\ \text{tab}}{500\ \cancel{\text{mg}}} \quad \Bigg| \quad 1500\ \cancel{\text{mg}} \quad = \quad \frac{1500}{500} \quad = \quad \textbf{3 tabs}$$

It is wise to **reduce** numbers prior to the multiplication step. This helps to decrease large numbers that will be multiplied and simplifies the problem. This is helpful when problems become more complex and contain more factors. For example:

$$?\text{tab} \quad = \quad \frac{1\ \text{tab}}{\underset{1}{\cancel{500}\ \cancel{\text{mg}}}} \quad \Bigg| \quad \overset{3}{\cancel{1500}\ \cancel{\text{mg}}} \quad = \quad \frac{3}{1} \quad = \quad \textbf{3 tabs}$$

8. **Ask: "Does this answer make sense?"**

(Continued)

REVIEW SHEET
DIMENSIONAL ANALYSIS CALCULATIONS *(cont'd)*

Using dimensional analysis for dosage calculations is particularly valuable when the nurse must convert between systems of measurement.

The physician has ordered the thyroid hormone levothyroxine (Synthroid), 0.1 mg PO for the patient. The pharmacist states that levothyroxine 50 mcg = 1 tablet is in stock.

1.   **Identify the final answer label.**

     State, **"The final answer to this dosage calculation will be labeled, "tablets" (tabs).**

     Ask, **"How many tablets will need to be administered to this patient?"**

     Write this question in abbreviated form to the far left of the calculation paper.

?tab =

2.   **Draw a grid.**

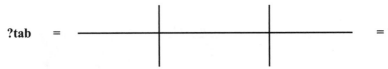

3.   **Find a given factor in the dosage calculation problem that is labeled with the same name as the final answer label.** Begin the process with the dosage relationships that are already known. In the above example, the physician has ordered a total of **0.1 mg** of the drug and the pharmacy has **tablets** of **50 micrograms (mcg)** each.

?tab   =   <u>1 tab</u>   =

4.   **Write the numbers in the problem in the correct form that shows a relationship or ratio.** In this case, it is given that 1 tablet contains 50 mcg of levothyroxine; in other words, 50 mcg per 1 tab is available. So, with the label of 1 tab above the grid line, the corresponding term of "50 mcg" is written below the line. This indicates the relationship or ratio of 1 tab to 50 mcg.

?tab   =   <u>1 tab</u>   =
        50 mcg

5.   **Check for a given factor with the same label that appears in the first, lower space or denominator position on the grid. Place the number that belongs with this unit label that in the next upper (numerator) space of the grid.**

     The answer to this drug calculation problem is the number of tablets that will equal the physician's ordered dose of 0.1 mg.

(Continued)

REVIEW SHEET
DIMENSIONAL ANALYSIS CALCULATIONS *(cont'd)*

There is a missing link in the problem because the drug available is labeled in micrograms (mcg) and the dosage desired is labeled in milligrams (mg). Placement of the unit labeled "mg" in the next upper space would not allow for cancellation. A conversion from mcg to mg is necessary to fill in that missing link.

$$?\text{tab} \quad = \quad \frac{1\ \text{tab}}{50\ \text{mcg}} \quad \bigg|\quad \frac{0.1\ \text{mg}}{} \quad\bigg|\quad \frac{0.1\ \text{mg}}{} \quad =$$

$$?\text{tab} \quad = \quad \frac{1\ \text{tab}}{50\ \text{mcg}} \quad\bigg|\quad \frac{1000\ \text{mcg}}{1\ \text{mg}} \quad\bigg|\quad \frac{0.1\ \text{mg}}{} \quad =$$

6. **Cancel Labels**.

$$?\text{tab} \quad = \quad \frac{1\ \text{tab}}{50\ \cancel{\text{mcg}}} \quad\bigg|\quad \frac{1000\ \cancel{\text{mcg}}}{1\ \cancel{\text{mg}}} \quad\bigg|\quad \frac{0.1\ \cancel{\text{mg}}}{} \quad =$$

7. **Calculate**. Reduce numbers if needed. Do this where possible in order to reduce the large numbers that need to be multiplied and divided.

$$?\text{tab} \quad = \quad \frac{1\ \text{tab}}{\overset{}{\underset{1}{\cancel{50}}}\ \cancel{\text{mcg}}} \quad\bigg|\quad \frac{\overset{20}{\cancel{1000}}\ \cancel{\text{mcg}}}{1\ \cancel{\text{mg}}} \quad\bigg|\quad \frac{0.1\ \cancel{\text{mg}}}{} \quad = \quad \frac{2}{1} \quad = \quad \textbf{2 tabs}$$

8. **Ask: "Does this answer make sense?"**

(Continued)

REVIEW SHEET
DIMENSIONAL ANALYSIS CALCULATIONS *(cont'd)*

How does dimensional analysis work if the answer needs to be labeled with more than one term, such as milliliters per hour (ml/hr) or drops per minute (gtt/min)? These are common answer labels when the nurse is calculating IV rates.

A patient has sustained a life-threatening hemorrhage. The physician orders 1000 mL of lactated Ringer's IV solution to be infused at 80 gtt/minute. The drop factor is 10 gtt = 1 mL. The nurse must set the IV pump to milliliters per hours. How many milliliters per hour will be infused?

1. **Identify the final answer label(s).**

   State, **"The final answer to this dosage calculation will be labeled 'milliliters per hour (mL/hr)'."**

   Ask, **"How many mL/hr need to be administered to this patient?"**

   Write this question in abbreviated form to the far left of the calculation paper.

   $$?\text{mL/hr} \;=$$

2. **Draw a grid.**

   $$?\text{mL/hr} \;=\; \frac{\quad\quad\quad|\quad\quad\quad}{\quad\quad\quad|\quad\quad\quad}\;=$$

3. **Find a given factor in the dosage calculation problem that is labeled with the same name as the top answer label.** It does not have to match the bottom label at this point.

   $$?\text{mL/hr} \;=\; \frac{1\text{ mL}\quad|\quad\quad}{\quad\quad|\quad\quad}\;=$$

4. **Write the numbers in the problem in the correct form that shows a relationship or ratio.** First, place those factors that exist in a relationship or ratio in the grid. In this case, place the relationship 1 mL = 10 gtts first.

   $$?\text{mL/hr} \;=\; \frac{\dfrac{1\text{ mL}}{10\text{ gtts}}\quad|\quad\quad}{\quad|\quad\quad}\;=$$

5. **Check for the given factor with the same unit label that appears in the first, lower space or denominator position on the grid.** Place the number that belongs with this label that in the next upper (numerator) space of the grid. Place the corresponding number and label in the grid below.

   $$?\text{mL/hr} \;=\; \dfrac{1\text{ mL}}{10\text{ gtts}}\;\bigg|\;\dfrac{80\text{ gtts}}{1\text{ min}}\;\bigg|\;=$$

(Continued)

REVIEW SHEET
DIMENSIONAL ANALYSIS CALCULATIONS *(cont'd)*

The answer needs to be in mL/hr and, if the calculation is performed at this point, the final answer will appear as mL/min. A conversion factor must be entered as follows:

$$\text{?mL/hr} \quad = \quad \frac{1 \text{ mL}}{10 \text{ gtts}} \quad \bigg| \quad \frac{80 \text{ gtts}}{1 \text{ min}} \quad \bigg| \quad \frac{60 \text{ min}}{1 \text{ hr}} \quad =$$

Examine the problem for the necessary numbers needed for calculation – ignore those that are not needed (extraneous) to arrive at the correct answer. There is one remaining factor in this calculation problem that has not been included in the grid. Through reasoning, the nurse knows that the 1000 mL factor is not necessary to calculate the mL/hr rate. Should there be some doubt as whether or not to use this number in a calculation, the fact that there is no logical place for it on the dimensional analysis grid provides a tip that it is not needed in the calculation for the answer of mL/hr.

6.   **Cancel Labels**. In this problem, labels that remain after cancellation are mL and hr indicating that the final answer will be labeled correctly.

$$\text{?mL/hr} \quad = \quad \frac{1 \text{ mL}}{10 \text{ gtts}} \quad \bigg| \quad \frac{80 \text{ gtts}}{1 \text{ min}} \quad \bigg| \quad \frac{60 \text{ min}}{1 \text{ hr}} \quad =$$

7. **Calculate**. Reduce numbers if needed.

$$\text{?mL/hr} \quad = \quad \frac{1 \text{ mL}}{10 \text{ gtts}} \quad \bigg| \quad \frac{80 \text{ gtts}}{1 \text{ min}} \quad \bigg| \quad \frac{60 \text{ min}}{1 \text{ hr}} \quad = \quad \frac{480}{1} \quad = \quad \frac{480 \text{ mL}}{1 \text{ hr}}$$

8.   **Ask: "Does this answer make sense?"**

In this case, 480 mL/hr is a large amount of fluid to infuse intravenously, and a nurse would correctly question the answer. However, the problem indicated that replacement of a significant intravascular deficit was necessary, so the answer does make sense.

WORKSHEET 9-7   Mastering Dimensional Analysis

Problem 1

The physician has ordered aspirin (ASA) gr 10 PO every 3 hours prn. The bottle says 325 mg = 1 tablet.

1. Identify the final answer label.

?tab =

2. Draw a grid.

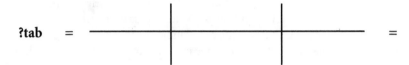

3. Find a given factor in the dosage calculation problem that is labeled with the same name as the final answer label.

?tab   =   ———————┼———————┼———————   =

4. Write the numbers in the problem in the correct form that shows a relationship or ratio.

?tab   =   ———————┼———————┼———————   =

5. Check for a given factor with the same label that appears in the first, lower space or denominator position on the grid. Place the number that belongs with this unit label that in the next upper (numerator) space of the grid.

?tab   =   ———————┼———————┼———————   =

6. Cancel labels.

?tab   =   ———————┼———————┼———————   =

7. Calculate.

?tab   =   ———————┼———————┼———————   =

8. Ask: "Does this answer make sense?"

(Continued)

WORKSHEET 9-7 Mastering Dimensional Analysis *(cont'd)*

Problem 2

A physician orders morphine sulfate gr 1/8 IM every 4 hours prn for postoperative pain. The bottle reads 15 mg/mL.

1. Identify the final answer label.

? mL =

2. Draw a grid.

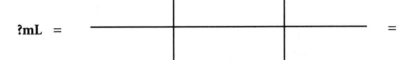

?mL =   =

3. Find a given factor in the dosage calculation problem that is labeled with the same name as the final answer label.

?mL =   =

4. Write the numbers in the problem in the correct form that shows a relationship or ratio.

?mL =   =

5. Check for a given factor with the same label that appears in the first, lower space, or denominator position, on the grid. Place the number that belongs with this unit label that in the next upper (numerator) space of the grid.

?mL =   =

6. Cancel labels.

?mL =   =

7. Calculate.

?mL =   =

8. Ask: "Does this answer make sense?"

10 Preparing and Administering Medications

Answer Key: A complete answer key was provided for your instructor.

OBJECTIVES

1. Compare dosage forms for drugs given by the enteral route.
2. Outline procedures for giving medications enterally, parenterally, and percutaneously.
3. Identify anatomy landmarks used for giving parenteral medications.
4. List processes to prevent human immunodeficiency virus (HIV) transmission.

Be sure to check out the bonus material on the free CD-ROM in your textbook, including:

Audio Pronunciation Guide
NCLEX®-Style Review Questions: Chapter 10
Video Clips
- Oral Medication
- Rectal Suppositories
- Medication from Ampule
- Medication from Vial
- Intradermal Medications
- Subcutaneous Injections
- Intramuscular Injections
- Initiating a Peripheral IV
- Topical Medications
- Measured Ointment
- Transdermal Patch
- Ear Drops
- Eye Drops
- Metered-Dose Inhaler

WORKSHEET 10-1   Recognizing Different Oral Dosage Forms

Match the following words with the proper descriptions.

Capsules	Elixirs	Emulsions	Lozenges
Suspensions	Syrups	Tablets	

1. A liquid with a high sugar content to disguise the bitter taste.

   _____

2. A dried powder compressed into small pellets.

   _____

3. A medication that is sucked.

   _____

4. A liquid that you shake prior to pouring.

   _____

5. A medication with a high alcohol content.

   _____

6. Gelatin containers that must not be opened or crushed.

   _____

7. A medication that contains an agent to increase the solubility.

   _____

8. A form that contains little medication compared to other ingredients.

   _____

9. This often forms the base of cough syrups.

   _____

10. A medication that comes in variety of colors and shapes and should not be broken.

   _____

11. A medication often given by the tablespoon; a more accurate dosage is not needed.

   _____

WORKSHEET 10-2   Problems with IV Infusions

Identify the mechanism causing the following problems with IV infusions and the nursing action needed to correct the problem.

1. Ms. Jones calls you because her IV is not running well. She has just returned from the bathroom, and the IV bottle is lying on the bed.

2. Mr. Harry mentions that after his bed bath, his arm began burning where the IV is inserted.

3. Terry Brown, age 3, has begun to cry, pulling at his arm. The IV infusion site is reddened.

4. Ms. Wizer is a very emaciated patient with gastric cancer. She has been receiving IVs for days. Today she is very restless and a little confused. She keeps putting on her light but doesn't really complain of anything when the nurse arrives. She just lies there gasping.

5. The alarm on the IV infusion pump for Mr. King begins to sound. You enter the room and find air in the tubing.

6. Ms. Wallace is a very obese patient with a broken hip. She is unable to get out of bed. You notice that her IV is not dripping. What would you check first?

7. Ms. Watson calls you into the room. She asks for another blanket because she has suddenly begun to shiver. She has 1 unit of blood running.

WORKSHEET 10-3   Working with Percutaneous Products

For each of the following percutaneous medications, indicate at least one thing that is important in administering medications to the appropriate site.

Ointment

Metered-dose inhaler

Lotion

Ear drops

Vaginal suppository

Nebulizer

Eyedrops

Patch

Shampoo

WORKSHEET 10-4   Working with Standard Precautions

Mr. Green was brought to the emergency room by the emergency medical technicians (EMTs). He was found in an alley in a highly intoxicated and confused state and has a large lump on his head. While you are helping Mr. Green move to an x-ray table he suddenly becomes incontinent of feces, which gets all over your clothing and arms.

Multiple Choice

1. How would you evaluate your risk of exposure to HIV or hepatitis B virus?
    1. Very high because your skin came into direct contact with feces
    2. Low for HIV, but very high for hepatitis B virus
    3. Very low because HIV and hepatitis B virus are blood-borne pathogens
    4. Low because the exposure to feces was not very extensive

2. Mr. Green begins to vomit. The vomitus is clear with streaks of bright red blood. Does this change your evaluation of risk?
    1. No, the gastric juices inactivate the HIV and hepatitis B virus.
    2. No, vomitus is not an implicated fluid for HIV or hepatitis B.
    3. No, vomitus is not potentially infectious in this situation.
    4. Yes, the contamination of vomitus with blood increases the risk of HIV or hepatitis B infection.

3. You just gave Mr. Green an antibiotic by injection. What special precautions will you take?
    1. Recap the needle and dispose of it in a puncture-resistant container located in patient's room.
    2. Use gloves when giving the injection. Dispose of the needle in a puncture-resistant container located in the patient's room.
    3. Make certain to bend the needle so that it cannot be used again.
    4. Wash your hands with soap and water before and after giving the injection.

4. Mr. Green has had numerous past admissions. When the old chart arrives you find that he does have a positive test for HIV. How will this affect you care for this patient?
    1. You wear gloves and protective barriers when performing procedures that may produce blood, take precautions to prevent injuries from needles, and wash hands and surfaces immediately with warm soap and water if they are contaminated with blood or other body fluids.
    2. You refuse to care for him because you do not want any further exposure to HIV.
    3. You wear gloves, mask, and gown whenever you enter the room.
    4. You do not need to take any special precautions with him, except to wear a gown.

5. In giving Mr. Green his next dose of antibiotic, you accidentally stick yourself with the needle. You should
    1. immediately scrub the area vigorously with pHisoHex and leave for the day.
    2. wash the area and fill out an incident report for the nursing supervisor.
    3. wash the area and follow the institution's procedure for reporting the incident and follow-up treatment.
    4. wash the area. You were giving an antibiotic so the risk of any infection to you is very small. Your institutional policy makes it optional whether you report it or not.

WORKSHEET 10-5 Ethical-Legal Situations to Ponder in Preparing and Administering Medications

1. Nurse Fairland has been preparing some Demerol for Mr. Jones, a patient who is in pain. Another of her patients is just returning from surgery and needs to be put to bed. Nurse Fairland asks you to give Mr. Jones the pain medication she has just drawn up while she helps the patient returning from surgery. How does this make you feel? What will you do?

2. You have worked on this medical unit for weeks and know all of the patients well. When you begin to give medications, you notice that Mr. Glenn isn't wearing an identification bracelet. He is elderly and confused, but you know him well. Is his missing ID bracelet a problem?

3. You arrive in Mrs. Babcock's room just as her husband comes to visit. Mrs. Babcock wants to walk in the hallway and asks you to leave her Lanoxin on the bedside table. "I'll take it when I get back!" she says. What will you do?

4. You accidentally stuck yourself with a needle after giving a patient an injection. What do you do? No one saw this happen. Does this affect what you would do? Why?

REVIEW SHEET
READING DRUG LABELS

Drug labels are required on all medication containers. The label must indicate the contents and the directions for its administration. When medications are packaged in the unit dose system, only one dose is provided in each package. The medication is not removed from the packaging until the medication is given to the patient.

By law, the drug label is required to list the following types of information:

- Drug name
- Dosage strength
- Formulation of medication: tablet, capsule, etc.
- Total amount per bottle or vial
- Manufacturer
- Instructions for storage or reconstitution
- Expiration date

Look at the following label:

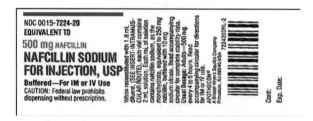

When only one name is listed—for example, NAFCILLIN SODIUM—this indicates a generic name. If there were a trade name listed on *this* label, nafcillin sodium would be listed in a smaller type underneath the trade name.

The drug label says for injection and further states that it is for IV or IM use. This makes it clear that it cannot be given orally.

The drug label also states that this is 500 mg nafcillin. The small type indicates the dosage per mL when the product is reconstituted and lists the usual adult dosage.

WORKSHEET 10-6   Practice in Reading Drug Labels

Look at the following labels and determine:

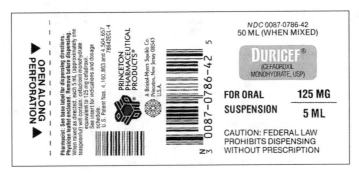

1. What are the generic and trade names of the medication?

2. How is this product to be administered?

3. What is the total mL in the bottle when mixed?

4. What is the dosage/mL when mixed?

5. Who is the manufacturer?

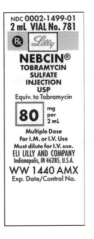

1. What are the generic and trade names of the medication?

2. Who is the manufacturer?

3. What is the total mL in the bottle?

4. What is the dosage per mL?

5. What other important information is provided?

(Continued)

WORKSHEET 10-6   Practice in Reading Drug Labels *(cont'd)*

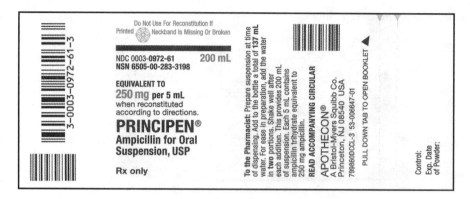

1. What are the generic and trade names of the drug?

2. What is the dosage/mL?

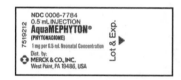 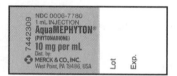

1. What are the differences in these two medication labels?

2. If a newborn is to receive AquaMEPHYTON 1 mg immediately after delivery, which vial would be used?

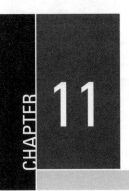

11 Allergy and Respiratory Medications

CHAPTER 11

Answer Key: A complete answer key was provided for your instructor.

OBJECTIVES

1. Identify major antihistamines used to treat breathing problems.
2. Describe the action of antitussive medications.
3. List medications used to treat and prevent asthma attacks.
4. Describe the major actions and the adverse reactions of the two main categories of bronchodilators.
5. Identify at least six medications commonly used as decongestants.
6. Describe the mechanism of action for expectorants.
7. List the major contraindications to the use of nasal steroids.

⚉ **Be sure to check out the bonus material on the free CD-ROM in your textbook, including:**

Audio Pronunciation Guide
NCLEX®-Style Review Questions: Chapter 11
Top 200 Drugs by Prescription

WORKSHEET 11-1   Antihistamines

1. Histamine, a chemical produced by the body,
   1. is released in response to mast cells and basophils.
   2. is released only when infection is present.
   3. produces the inflammatory response in the body.
   4. acts to relieve the erythema and swelling caused by inflammation.

2. Antihistamines act to competitively block
   1. the action of histamine by producing vasodilation and increased capillary permeability.
   2. histamine action by antagonizing vasodilation and increased capillary permeability.
   3. the action of acetylcholine by occupying the H_1 receptor sites at effector structures.
   4. the action of anticholinergic receptors in effector structures.

3. Seasonal allergic rhinitis refers to
   1. colds that develop only during Christmas season.
   2. a runny nose in the summer.
   3. a runny nose caused by perennial allergic phenomena.
   4. an allergy that develops during the holidays.

4. The adverse reaction most commonly associated with antihistamines is
   1. tachycardia.
   2. difficult urination.
   3. insomnia.
   4. sedation.

5. The concurrent use of CNS depressants with antihistamines would produce
   1. increased sedation.
   2. paradoxical excitation.
   3. urinary retention.
   4. tachycardia.

6. Evaluation of a patient with seasonal allergic rhinitis might reveal
   1. the presence of a productive cough.
   2. swollen, pale nasal mucosa and clear, watery nasal discharge.
   3. red, swollen nasal turbinates, and thick, greenish discharge.
   4. crackles in the lungs and wheezes on expiration.

7. Antihistamines should be used in young children
   1. if the family has a history of sleep apnea.
   2. if the child has symptoms of Reye's syndrome.
   3. cautiously, if at all.
   4. with one large dose at bedtime.

True/False

8. T   F   All antihistamines are available over the counter.
9. T   F   Antihistamines are relatively safe, and most patients will not have trouble with them.
10. T   F   If tolerance to one type of antihistamine develops, switching to another type may restore responsiveness.
11. T   F   Rebound effect means that the patient quickly bounces back and recovers from the problem.
12. T   F   Antihistamines frequently produce gastrointestinal side effects.

WORKSHEET 11-2   Antitussives

1. Antitussive agents are used to
   1. promote expectoration.
   2. prevent a cough from developing.
   3. thin the secretions in the bronchial airways.
   4. relieve coughing.

2. Narcotic antitussives act by
   1. anesthetizing the stretch receptors in the medulla.
   2. reducing the cough at its source in the respiratory passages.
   3. acting peripherally in the pleura.
   4. suppressing the cough reflex by acting directly on the cough center in the brain.

3. Antitussive agents are used primarily in
   1. patients who cannot sleep or work due to severe productive cough and fever.
   2. patients with a productive cough that is associated with pneumonia.
   3. nonproductive coughs.
   4. chronic allergic conditions.

4. The most common adverse reactions to antitussives include
   1. drowsiness, dry mouth, and tachycardia.
   2. drowsiness, muscle aches, and high blood pressure.
   3. constipation; dry mouth; and dry, cracked mucosa.
   4. drowsiness, dry mouth, nausea, and postural hypotension.

True/False

5. T   F   If a narcotic antitussive is given with a CNS depressant, a reduced dosage should be used.
6. T   F   Antitussives are often administered to patients with chronic pulmonary disease.
7. T   F   The amount of narcotic in these antitussive products is very small, and there is almost no risk of producing drug dependence in a patient.
8. T   F   Antitussives may cause dizziness when patients get up from a lying or sitting position.
9. T   F   Antitussive medications are all available over the counter.
10. T   F   Narcotic antitussive medications frequently produce constipation.

11. Antitussives are often combined with other medications in order to
    1. appeal to the patient who is buying an over-the-counter medication.
    2. make it easier for the patient by avoiding having to take several pills.
    3. reduce the chances for medication errors.
    4. reduce the cost of buying separate medications.

12. One of the most important things to teach a patient taking an antitussive medication would be
    1. to take the medication as ordered by the physician; not to alter the dosage or frequency.
    2. to drink lots of orange juice or water while taking this drug.
    3. that the medication may cause drowsiness or nausea.
    4. to take the drug with food or milk to decrease stomach upset.

WORKSHEET 11-3   Medications Used in the Treatment of Asthma and COPD

1. What is the physiologic result of bronchospasm?
   1. More mucus is produced in the respiratory tract.
   2. Narrowing of the lumen restricts the amount of air that is pulled into or pulled out of the lungs with each breath.
   3. Vasodilation is produced sympathetically.
   4. Bronchodilation results.

2. The two major types of bronchodilators are
   1. theophylline and xanthines.
   2. sympathomimetics and adrenergics.
   3. sympathomimetics and xanthine derivatives.
   4. beta$_2$ adrenergics and anticholinergics.

3. Sympathomimetics relax bronchial smooth muscle by
   1. stimulation of beta$_2$-adrenergic receptors.
   2. stimulation of alpha-adrenergic receptors.
   3. stimulation of beta$_1$-adrenergic receptors.
   4. blockade of direct stimulation of smooth muscles.

4. The vasopressor response throughout the body produces vasoconstriction in blood vessels of the bronchial mucosa, which results in
   1. reduction of edema in the mucosa and submucosal tissue of the respiratory tract.
   2. increased myocardial contractility and condition.
   3. increased swelling and mucosal edema.
   4. increased mucus production and ciliary paralysis.

5. Common adverse effects of the sympathomimetics include
   1. increased heart rate, anorexia, restlessness, and insomnia.
   2. drowsiness, slow heart rate, and respiratory depression.
   3. polyuria, increased appetite, and hypertension.
   4. anorexia, nausea, vomiting, constipation, and diarrhea.

6. One of the major drawbacks of adrenergic bronchodilators is that
   1. their action often produces severe adverse reactions.
   2. drug interactions are present with most drugs.
   3. their effects are not limited to beta$_2$-type receptors.
   4. they have only local effects.

7. Sympathomimetic bronchodilators may be given by all routes of administration, except
   1. orally.
   2. via IPPB nebulizers.
   3. rectally.
   4. parenterally.

8. When sympathomimetic bronchodilators appear to be ineffective, the patient might
   1. use two different types of sympathomimetics at the same time.
   2. alternate two different sympathomimetic drugs.
   3. stop taking the medication, because an infection may be present.
   4. report the problem to the physician immediately.

9. Refractoriness is
   1. often caused by too frequent administration of drugs.
   2. infrequent with these products.
   3. caused when the underlying condition worsens.
   4. often related to food-drug interactions.

(Continued

ORKSHEET 11-3   Medications Used in the Treatment of Asthma and COPD *(cont'd)*

Mr. Jones complains of cough, a tickling sensation in his throat, and sneezing following use of his aerosol nebulizer. The nurse should tell him that this
1. is common and indicates the medication is getting down into the lungs where it is designed to work well.
2. is caused by bronchial irritation.
3. reflects the beginning of an allergic reaction.
4. response is caused by the oxygen propellant in the aerosol.

Paradoxical bronchospasm is a condition in which constriction of the lumen
1. becomes intermittent.
2. develops just prior to the use of bronchodilators.
3. develops following the use of bronchodilators.
4. alternates with bronchodilation.

Mr. Allen complains that the bronchodilators keep him from falling asleep at night. You might suggest
1. taking the medication with a glass of warm milk at bedtime.
2. taking a glass of alcohol to help relax before going to bed.
3. taking medication several hours before going to bed.
4. asking the physician for a mild sedative to counteract the effects of the bronchodilator.

The major differences in action between sympathomimetics and xanthine derivatives is that
1. xanthine derivatives produce significant CNS effects.
2. xanthine derivatives act directly on smooth muscle to achieve bronchial constriction.
3. xanthine derivatives do not have the systemic effects that sympathomimetics produce.
4. sympathomimetics also act directly on the kidney to produce diuresis.

Miss Laney has been in the emergency room with an asthma attack for 3 hours. She has been receiving a parenteral infusion containing aminophylline. She continues to wheeze and now begins to complain of nausea. The nurse should
1. let the physician know that the patient is not responding.
2. let the physician know that the patient is getting worse.
3. tell the patient that this is very common.
4. alert the physician to a possible adverse reaction.

Chris is a 9-year-old boy who takes Theo-Dur regularly to control asthma symptoms. He has been playing in a soccer game today and came into the clinic because of constant coughing. You find that his pulse is irregular. You determine that
1. vigorous exercise commonly causes an irregular pulse in children.
2. overdosage with xanthine products often produces ventricular dysrhythmias.
3. his symptoms probably indicate a need for increased medication.
4. the patient may have developed a respiratory infection and the exertion of playing soccer has caused the cardiac irregularity.

The half-life of xanthine bronchodilators is influenced by which of the following specific factors?
1. The age of the patient
2. The severity of the bronchospasm
3. Whether the patient smokes
4. The state of hydration of the patient

Monitoring the correct dosage of xanthine products is best accomplished by
1. decreasing the dose, if the patient begins vomiting.
2. determining if the frequency of prn medication use is increasing.
3. monitoring symptom relief.
4. obtaining the theophylline blood level.

(Continued)

WORKSHEET 11-3   Medications Used in the Treatment of Asthma and COPD *(cont'd)*

18. Factors that do not affect the blood levels of theophylline include
    1. the age of the patient.
    2. varying the theophylline-base content in different products.
    3. the metabolism and excretion of each drug.
    4. the sex of the patient.

True/False
19. T   F   The theophylline-base content varies in xanthine products.
20. T   F   The rate of absorption of oral theophylline depends on the dosage form used.
21. T   F   Enteric-coated or sustained-release tablets and capsules produce inconsistent blood levels.
22. T   F   Oral liquids have the fastest absorption time.
23. T   F   Food does not influence absorption of theophylline.
24. T   F   Rectal solutions and IM administration are closely equal to oral solutions in rate of absorption.
25. T   F   Metabolism and excretion time of theophylline varies.

26. Cromolyn sodium is a medication used for
    1. acute treatment of severe asthma attacks.
    2. acute COPD relapse.
    3. prophylaxis of asthma attacks.
    4. acute treatment of exertional asthma.

27. In using a cromolyn spinhaler patients should
    1. blow out as hard as possible when using the spinhaler.
    2. make certain to rinse the spinhaler in warm water after each treatment.
    3. stop using the spinhaler if it causes coughing each time it is used.
    4. carry the spinhaler with them so it can be used if they have a sudden asthma attack.

28. Leukotriene receptor inhibitors are used primarily to
    1. block bronchospasm.
    2. reduce inflammation.
    3. thin mucus secretions.
    4. dilate bronchioles.

29. Systemic corticosteroids are used primarily for the purpose of
    1. enhancing the action of cromolyn sodium.
    2. decreasing the inflammatory activity in the bronchioles in acute asthma attacks and enhancing the ac-
       tivity of other drugs.
    3. producing direct smooth muscle constriction.
    4. decreasing the effect of beta-adrenergic drugs

30. Use of systemic corticosteroids in asthma is reserved for
    1. severe episodes of asthma that do not respond to other drugs.
    2. short-term therapy only.
    3. solo drug therapy only.
    4. patients with no other systemic problems.

WORKSHEET 11-4   Decongestants

What is the main action of decongestants?

Define rebound vasodilation.

Decongestants are used for the relief of nasal congestion caused by:

_____ and _____ secondary to mucosal dryness sometimes follow topical administration of decongestants.

Rebound congestion is often seen following:

Decongestants are contraindicated in patients with:

Topical decongestants should be used only in _____ cases, for no longer than _____, and sparingly in _____ and the _____.

(Continued)

WORKSHEET 11-4   Decongestants *(cont'd)*

8. _____ decongestants are considered more effective than _____ preparations because they will produce effects in _____.

9. What is the disadvantage of the systemic oral decongestant?

10. What is the advantage of topical application of decongestant?

11. Identify one disadvantage of nasal drops.

12. Why must care be used when instilling nasal drops?

13. _____ are often marketed to appeal to the patient with a wide variety of symtoms who is buying an _____ medication.

WORKSHEET 11-5   Expectorants

Expectorant products are believed to act by:

There are _____ objective studies to support the clinical effectiveness of these drugs.

These products are used in the _____ of _____ cough.

Identify the most common adverse reaction to expectorant.

Which expectorant may increase bleeding tendency as a drug interaction with anticoagulants?

When are expectorants not to be used?

Chronic or persistent cough may be the result of:

Thick, tenacious mucus may be reduced by taking expectorants and:

What specific instructions would you give the patient about drinking liquids?

. Use this medication dose _____ in order to decrease the risk of
_____.

WORKSHEET 11-6   Intranasal Steroids

1. The main action of intranasal steroids is
    1. increasing the local blood supply in the nasal mucosa.
    2. stimulation of the inflammatory response.
    3. beta-stimulation of adrenergic receptors.
    4. suppression of the inflammatory reaction.

2. Intranasal steroids are used in the treatment of _____, _____, and _____ induced nasal inflammation; or _____.

3. When are topical nasal steroids used?

4. Identify the most common adverse reactions to intranasal steroids.

5. In comparing the intranasal steroids to systemic steroids, in general the nasal steroids may be said to have:

6. Steroids pose a risk in their use because the drug may:

7. The patient should be observed for signs of systemic absorption since _____ and _____ may develop.

8. The patient should be cautioned to _____ and not _____, especially if large doses have been used for long periods of time.

◆ Chapter 11—Integrated Case Studies ◆

Case One

Lisa Fines, 28 years old, comes to the clinic with a clear nasal discharge, red itchy eyes, and a cough of 3 days' duration.

.   What other important information would you like to obtain from her history?

.   What information would you like to obtain from the physical examination?

.   What pattern of subjective and objective findings would make you believe she had seasonal allergic rhinitis? Asthma? A URTI?

.   What would be the difference in treatment for seasonal allergic rhinitis, asthma, or a URTI?

.   Would there be any modifications in the recommended treatment if Lisa were pregnant? A child or only 2 years of age? An elderly patient with congestive heart failure?

(Continued)

◆ Chapter 11—Integrated Case Studies *(cont'd)* ◆

Case Two

Mrs. Plains is a 43-year-old African American woman who reports wheezing and tightness in her chest since early this morning. She went shopping today and has been outside during an unseasonable cold spell, which she believes is the cause of the wheezing. She has had one other episode of wheezing that occurred 3 days ago while she was outside in the cold. She has a slight cough that is productive of a small amount of clear sputum. For the last 3 or 4 days she has awakened at night, particularly early in the morning, with dyspnea and a cough. She has no other symptoms.

> **Physical examination:** Afebrile and in no acute distress.
> **Cardiovascular:** Heart rate 84 beats/min, blood pressure 114/84 mm Hg.
> **Respiratory:** Breath sounds equal throughout both sides; scattered monophonic expiratory wheezes throughout lung fields.

1. The physician decides that Mrs. Plains has a moderately persistent, reversible airway obstruction that is responsive to bronchodilators and corticosteroids. She is started on an oral inhaler. What might the doctor order? Give the name, dosage, frequency, and patient instructions for each medication you select.

	Name	Dosage	Frequency	Patient Instructions
a.				
b.				
c.				

2. Mrs. Plains comes back in 1 month. Two weeks ago she had a cold with nasal congestion, sneezing, and a sore throat. Since then, the cough has worsened and she is now producing large amounts of purulent sputum. What do you think has happened?

3. The physician orders erythromycin EES one tablet PO three times daily. Why?

4. Mrs. Plains returns 1 month later. Her cough and sputum production have resolved. She continues to have wheezing when she goes out in the cold. What self-management plans would you discuss with her?

CHAPTER 12 — Antiinfective Medications

Answer Key: A complete answer key was provided for your instructor.

OBJECTIVES

1. Identify the major antiinfective drug categories and the organisms against which they are effective.
2. Define "spectrum" and explain what this word means in antiinfective therapy.
3. List some of the most common adverse reactions to medications used to treat infections.
4. Outline the most important things to teach the patient who is taking antiinfective medications.

Be sure to check out the bonus material on the free CD-ROM in your textbook, including:

Audio Pronunciation Guide
NCLEX®-Style Review Questions: Chapter 12
Top 200 Drugs by Prescription

WORKSHEET 12-1   Penicillins

1. Penicillin is the drug of choice in:

2. The choice of drug is dependent on:

3. Name at least three organisms against which penicillin is commonly effective.

4. Identify the most common adverse reactions.

5. What is the most severe form of adverse reaction?

6. Drug interactions may be summarized as:

7. Different classifications of penicillin include:

8. What specific instructions do you give the patient regarding the duration of penicillin therapy?

9. What problems may develop as a result of inadequate duration of treatment with penicillin?

WORKSHEET 12-2   Sulfonamides

1. Name at least three acute or chronic infections in which the sulfonamides are commonly used.

2. Name one common preoperative use for sulfonamides.

3. What special questions must be asked while taking the history of a patient in whom sulfonamides might be used?

4. What are some adverse reactions to sulfonamides?

5. What is the one adverse reaction that can often be reduced with proper patient education?

6. What are some of the potentially serious adverse reactions for which the nurse and patient must watch?

(Continued)

WORKSHEET 12-2   Sulfonamides *(cont'd)*

7. Indicate the effect that concurrent use of these medications would have on a sulfonamide product.

Medication	Effect of Concurrent Use
Oral anticoagulants	_____
Probenecid	_____
Thiazide diuretics	_____
Salicylates	_____
Indomethacin	_____
Penicillin	_____
Antacids	_____
Phenytoin	_____
Uricosuric agents	_____

8. Medication should be discontinued if _____ or
    _____.

9. The nurse needs to warn the patient about protecting:

10. What information must be included in specific teaching instructions to a patient taking a sulfonamide?

11. List at least three sulfonamide products, and indicate the routes by which they may be administered.

12. What is in a sulfonamide combination product, and why are these combinations used?

WORKSHEET 12-3   Broad-Spectrum Antibiotics

1. Broad-spectrum antibiotics commonly have two mechanisms of action. Describe them.

2. Antibiotics also may be considered either *bacterio-* _____ or *bacterio-* _____. Define these two terms.

3. Broad-spectrum antibiotics are used in the treatment of
   1. infective organisms.
   2. pathogenic organisms.
   3. susceptible organisms.

4. How is the appropriate antibiotic selected?

5. Bacterial organisms may be classified by _____ and
   _____.

6. An antibiotic with a broad spectrum of activity would be effective against:

7. The three types of major adverse reactions seen with antibiotic therapy include _____,
   and _____, _____.

8.   Superinfections are commonly caused by:

(Continued)

WORKSHEET 12-3   Broad-Spectrum Antibiotics *(cont'd)*

9. Identify the most common tissues adversely affected by antibiotic therapy.

10. Identify symptoms that may alert the nurse to the development of direct tissue damage.

_____

_____

True/False

11. T   F   True hypersensitivity reactions are uncommon.
12. T   F   Skin rash is a common allergic symptom.
13. T   F   Anasarca is the most serious form of hypersensitivity.
14. T   F   If a patient is allergic to penicillin, the drug of choice is often erythromycin.
15. T   F   If a patient develops hives, facial swelling, and general irritability, we say he has cross-sensitivity.

16. Describe clinically what to look for with anaphylaxis.

    What happens?

    When?

    Why?

(Continued)

WORKSHEET 12-3   Broad-Spectrum Antibiotics *(cont'd)*

17. In the following table, identify for each specific antibiotic the most important adverse reaction to monitor.

Antibiotic	Adverse Reaction to Monitor
chloramphenicol	
erythromycin	
clindamycin	
colistin	
lincomycin	
aminoglycosides	

True/False
18. T   F   Drug interactions with antibiotics are common.
19. T   F   All antibiotics should be taken with food or milk to decrease gastrointestinal upset.
20. T   F   Antibiotics rarely interfere with serum laboratory tests.
21. T   F   Most antibiotics do not cross the placental barrier and may be given to pregnant women.

WORKSHEET 12-4   Antitubercular Agents

1. What organism causes tuberculosis?

True/False

2. T   F   Tuberculosis is a disease rarely seen in the United States today.
3. T   F   Tuberculosis is a disease that is found only in the lungs of humans.
4. T   F   The drugs used in treating tuberculosis do not kill the bacterium but prevent its spread through the patient or to other individuals.
5. T   F   Antituberculosis medications prevent the bacterium from producing new cell walls.

6. Define antitubercular chemoprophylaxis.

7. Define antitubercular chemotherapy.

8. Individuals at high risk for developing tuberculosis include
    1. all children up to age 13.
    2. household members of those recently diagnosed with tuberculosis.
    3. individuals whose skin tests have become positive within the last 2 years.
    4. individuals with other debilitating disease.
    5. individuals with positive skin tests who are under 35 years of age.

9.   What is the biggest problem with administering antitubercular drugs over a longer period of time?

10. Many of the medications used to treat tuberculosis are associated with severe tissue damage to the:

(Continued)

WORKSHEET 12-4   Antitubercular Agents *(cont'd)*

11. An important consideration in administering antitubercular drugs is to avoid concurrent administration of any other drugs that may produce:

12. In order to help prevent the development of drug resistance, the plan of care should encourage monitoring what three things?

13. General characteristics of antitubercular therapy for active tuberculosis include
    1. giving one drug for active tuberculosis.
    2. giving several drugs for active tuberculosis.
    3. short-term drug therapy.
    4. long-term drug therapy.
    5. multiple dosing during the day.
    6. one-time daily dosing.
    7. parenteral medication only.
    8. oral medication only.

14. Most antitubercular medications cause gastric irritation and should be taken with food. Identify the one medication that is better absorbed on an empty stomach.

15. Identify the treatment of choice in chemotherapy for uncomplicated active pulmonary tuberculosis.

16. If a patient has been treated for tuberculosis previously and becomes symptomatic again, what should be suspected?

(Continued)

WORKSHEET 12-4   Antitubercular Agents *(cont'd)*

17. Use of isoniazid and pyrazinamide together may lead to the development of
_____ and the patient should be monitored for
_____.

18. Monitoring of treatment effectiveness includes the regular monitoring of:

19. Identify the drug of choice for adult tuberculosis prophylaxis. _____

How much should be taken?

How long should it be taken?

WORKSHEET 12-5   Antiparasitic Agents

1. What parasite causes amebiasis? _____

2. Identify the most common extraintestinal infection. _____

3. List the five major drugs used for the treatment of amebiasis.

4. List the common precautions or contraindications for the use of amebicides.

5. Identify the one amebicide known to cause significant drug interactions.

6. Why should patients receiving emetine live sedentary lifestyles during the time of treatment?

7. Selection of the appropriate anthelmintic must be based on:

8. Identify the drug of choice for different types of worms that follow.

    Cutaneous larva migrans _____

    Cestodiasis (tapeworms) _____

    Roundworms _____

    Hookworms _____

    Pinworms _____

    Wuchereria bancrofti filariasis _____

(Continued)

WORKSHEET 12-5   Antiparasitic Agents *(cont'd)*

9. Once the type of worm is identified, special instructions should be given to the patient about how to avoid spreading the infestation. These instructions include:

10. How may reinfection be prevented?

11. What does endemic mean?

12. What causes malaria?

13. Why is a variety of medications used in the treatment of malaria?

14. Antimalarial preparations are used for:

(Continued)

WORKSHEET 12-5   Antiparasitic Agents *(cont'd)*

15. What is cinchonism?

16. List the symptoms of cinchonism.

17. Patients on prolonged therapy or high doses of antimalarial products should be monitored closely for:

18. Why must patients taking quinine products be evaluated for cardiac dysrhythmias?

◆ Chapter 12—Integrated Case Study ◆

Bill Ethington, 64 years old, comes into the clinic with a temperature of 104° F. He is sweating profusely, feels nauseated, and says that he feels "horrible." He reports he has never felt this way before. He sits in the chair but twists and turns, rubbing his lower back as he talks. A urine specimen is positive for red blood cells and protein, and a microscopic specimen shows bacteria and urinary casts. The nurse practitioner confirms that he has a urinary tract infection.

1. What antibiotics are used primarily for urinary tract infections and why?

2. What special instructions would you give the patient if the nurse practitioner started the patient on Gantrisin?

3. What other problems does Mr. Ethington have that need nursing or medical care?

4. Would the medication ordered be any different if this patient was a pregnant woman?

5. What other types of drugs might Mr. Ethington need?

13 Antivirals, Antiretrovirals, and Antifungal Medications

Answer Key: A complete answer key was provided for your instructor.

OBJECTIVES

1. Describe how antiviral and antiretroviral medications work.
2. List common medications used in treating AIDS and AIDS-related fungal infections.
3. Outline Standard Precautions the nurse takes in limiting exposure to AIDS. (Review material in Chapter 10.)

Be sure to check out the bonus material on the free CD-ROM in your textbook, including:

Audio Pronunciation Guide
NCLEX®-Style Review Questions: Chapter 13
Top 200 Drugs by Prescription

WORKSHEET 13-1   Antiviral and Antiretroviral Medications

1. What is the difference between acquired immunodeficiency syndrome (AIDS) and human immunodeficiency virus (HIV)?

2. What are retroviruses?

3. What is the action of AIDS in the body?

4. If viral infections are not suppressed by antibiotics, why do we use these drugs in the treatment of patients with viral infections?

5. What viral conditions may be treated by medications?

6. Most antiviral products have significant toxicity associated with them. What are some of the more important problems?

(Continued)

WORKSHEET 13-1   Antiviral and Antiretroviral Medications *(cont'd)*

7. Name the two types of antiretroviral medications.

   a. _____

   b. _____

8. What is the purpose of using antiretroviral medications?

9. What tests are used to monitor the severity of disease and the effectiveness of AIDS treatment?

10. What is Crix Belly?

WORKSHEET 13-2   Antifungal Medications

1. What is a mycotic infection?

2. Fungi are found in two major forms in the body. Describe them.

3. List four commonly used fungicides.

4. What is the name of the organism that causes fungal vaginal infections in women and that is now seen so commonly in AIDS patients?

5. Adverse drug reactions produced by fungicides are
   1. associated with severe ototoxicity and hepatotoxicity.
   2. rare.
   3. generally mild, transient, and dosage-related.
   4. generally irritating but not very serious.

6. Severe superinfections may result with prolonged coadministration of fungicides with:

7. Assessment for signs or symptoms of superficial or vaginal fungal infection may demonstrate:

8. Evaluation of the patient taking fungicides would include:

◆ Chapter 13—Integrated Case Study ◆

Ms. Lucille Betts, a patient who has AIDS, comes into the clinic complaining of numbness and a burning sensation in her feet and lower legs. A physical examination shows her reflexes to be intact, but she has decreased sensation of light touch, pinprick, temperature, and vibration in the feet and midcalf. She has been under treatment with a reverse transcriptase inhibitor.

1. What do you believe is going on?

2. If the symptoms are ignored, what is the usual course?

3. What is the treatment?

4. Lucille discovers she is pregnant. What special requirements for treatment are there for pregnant women?

5. Lucille reports a thick white vaginal discharge and severe perineal itching. What is the probable diagnosis?

6. Why are infections of this type common in immunocompromised individuals?

(Continued)

◆ Chapter 13—Integrated Case Study *(cont'd)* ◆

7. What type of precautions should health care providers use in performing the vaginal examination on Lucille?

8. Lucille has an allergy to penicillin. Why might this be a problem for her?

9. Lucille is started on a vaginal antifungal medication. The nurse warns her that _____ is common skin reaction associated with many antifungal medications.

10. Most vaginal infections are cured within 3 to 4 days. Is there any reason to suspect that this will not be the case with Lucille?

11. Lucille is at risk for fungal infections at what other sites?

14 Antineoplastic Medications

Answer Key: A complete answer key was provided for your instructor.

OBJECTIVES

1. List the types of drugs used to treat neoplastic disease or cancer.
2. Identify the major adverse reactions associated with antineoplastic agents.
3. Develop a teaching plan for a patient taking an antineoplastic drug.

Be sure to check out the bonus material on the free CD-ROM in your textbook, including:

Audio Pronunciation Guide
NCLEX®-Style Review Questions: Chapter 14
Top 200 Drugs by Prescription

WORKSHEET 14-1 Antineoplastic Agents

Fill in the following chart describing antineoplastic drug actions.

Type of Antineoplastic Drug   **Action**

1. _____   Interfere with cell division

2. Antibiotics   _____

3. _____   Interfere with various metabolic functions

4. _____   Counteract effects of tumors dependent on male or female hormones

5. _____   Stop cell division directly

6. Antineoplastic agents may be used
   1. in place of radiation or surgery.
   2. in place of radiation.
   3. in place of surgery.
   4. before radiation or surgery.
   5. following radiation or surgery.

7. A term used to describe antineoplastic drug therapy is
   1. pharmacotherapy.
   2. radiotherapy.
   3. chemotherapy.
   4. physiotherapy.

8. Antineoplastic drug therapy is most likely to affect
   1. rapidly growing and dividing cells.
   2. only slow-growing cells spreading throughout the body.
   3. all cells of the body.
   4. only malignant cells.

(Continued)

WORKSHEET 14-1   Antineoplastic Agents *(cont'd)*

In addition to malignant cells, some normal cells in the body are commonly affected by antineoplastic agents. Fill in the following chart with the adverse reaction most likely to be produced when the cells listed are affected.

Normal Cells Attacked   **Adverse Reaction Seen**

9. GI tract   _____

10. Bone marrow   _____

11. Hair follicles   _____

12. Mouth   _____

13. Ovary or testes   _____

14. Antineoplastic medications are frequently given
    1. intravenously by the family at home.
    2. whenever needed during in-hospital stays.
    3. by the physician.
    4. only as a last resort when other measures have been unsuccessful.

15. Because patients with malignancies are often so fearful, it is important to remember that
    1. there is very little chance therapy will be helpful.
    2. the patient must be taught as much as possible about the problem and the therapy.
    3. it is important to conceal any bad news from the patient.
    4. medications are often helpful only when given intravenously as soon as the patient is diagnosed.

◆ Chapter 14—Integrated Case Study ◆

Bonnie Taylor, 48 years old, is admitted to the hospital with a diagnosis of acute lymphoblastic leukemia (ALL) and *Salmonella* sepsis. She has had four other admissions for chemotherapy and supportive care. She has lost weight and currently weighs 110 pounds. She is to receive platelets and a whole blood transfusion. The medications prescribed include:

> Acetaminophen (Tylenol) 650 mg PO q4h for fever.
> Gentamicin (Garamycin) 50 mg IV q8h.
> 6-Mercaptopurine (Purinethol) 200 mg PO daily.
> Trimethobenzamide HCl (Tigan) 200 mg suppository q6h prn.

1. The usual adult daily dose of 6-mercaptopurine is 2.5 mg/kg/day. How does this compare with what is ordered?

2. The usual adult daily dose of gentamicin is 3 mg/kg/day in three equal doses, given every 8 hours by IV. If the product comes in doses of 40 mg/mL, how much medication will be drawn up to be injected?

3. Why is gentamicin ordered?

4. Why is 6-mercaptopurine ordered?

5. Why is trimethobenzamide HCl ordered?

6. Why might this patient have an elevated temperature? What would you give her and when?

7. What other chemotherapeutic agents might be used for the treatment of leukemia?

8. Because of her condition and all of the medications she is taking, what are some of the things you would monitor?

15 Cardiovascular and Renal Medications

Answer Key: A complete answer key was provided for your instructor.

OBJECTIVES

1. Identify the approved way to give different forms of antianginal therapy.
2. Discuss the uses and general actions of cardiac drugs used to treat dysrhythmias.
3. Describe the common treatment for various types of lipoprotein disorders.
4. Explain the actions of different categories of drugs used to treat hypertension.
5. List the general uses and actions of cardiotonic drugs.
6. Identify indications for electrolyte replacement.

Be sure to check out the bonus material on the free CD-ROM in your textbook, including:

Audio Pronunciation Guide
NCLEX®-Style Review Questions: Chapter 15
Animations
- Normal Electrophysiology
- Renin-Angiotensin in Control of Blood Pressure
Top 200 Drugs by Prescription

WORKSHEET 15-1   Antianginals and Peripheral Vasodilators

1. How do vasodilators promote blood flow to the extremities?

2. What adverse reactions might be caused by nitroglycerin?

3. Are long-acting or short-acting nitrate products better in aborting an acute attack of angina? Why?

4. If a patient has developed a physiologic tolerance to nitroglycerin, should the dosage be increased to achieve pain relief?

5. Vasodilator medications relax the smooth muscles of peripheral arterial blood vessels. What action does this produce in the body?

6. What side effects are produced by peripheral vasodilating agents?

(Continued)

WORKSHEET 15-1   Antianginals and Peripheral Vasodilators *(cont'd)*

'. What action do nitrites have on coronary arteries? What is the benefit of this action on the heart?

. Do peripheral vasodilating agents affect the peripheral pulses of patients?

. Would nitrites be particularly useful in patients with intermittent claudication?

0. Should nitroglycerin ointment be massaged into the skin before covering with the dressing? Why or why not?

1. Mr. Stetson, age 69, experiences frequent attacks of angina pectoris. His blood pressure is elevated, and he has glaucoma. He is also a heavy beer drinker. Mr. Stetson
   1. should be started promptly on nitroglycerin.
   2. should be started on prophylactic therapy with long-acting nitrites.
   3. should not use nitroglycerin products.

2. Ms. Watson has been taking nitroglycerin to prevent anginal attacks. In assessing Ms. Watson before she leaves the hospital, you would check for
   1. skin rash, itching, or irritation at the patch site.
   2. the presence of epigastric distress, nausea, or vertigo.
   3. the presence of headache, or burning under her tongue with use of the medication.

3. Mr. Teldrin is recovering from an attack of angina. He will be leaving the hospital tomorrow. He has been instructed to take nitroglycerin sublingually if the anginal pain returns. You would give him which of the following additional instructions?
   1. During an attack of angina, he may repeat the dose after 5 to 10 minutes if the pain is not relieved.
   2. He can take as many tablets as necessary until relief is obtained.
   3. He should never repeat a dose but should call the physician immediately.
   4. If the pain is not relieved 5 minutes after taking the first dose, he should take a second dose. A third dose may be taken in another 5 minutes. If the pain is not relieved, he should go to an emergency room or doctor's office.

(Continued)

WORKSHEET 15-1   Antianginals and Peripheral Vasodilators *(cont'd)*

14. If a person does not receive relief from anginal pain after taking several nitroglycerin doses, you might suspect
    1. an allergy to the drug has developed.
    2. the nitroglycerin cannot relieve very severe pain.
    3. a larger dose is needed.
    4. the patient may be having a myocardial infarction.

15. Which of the following information would be shared with the patient and his family before discharge?
    1. Nitroglycerin tablets are narcotics used to relieve pain.
    2. A supply of nitroglycerin should be carried with the patient in a pill container and renewed every year.
    3. Nitroglycerin tablets may be refrigerated.
    4. Protect the tablets from damage by using the cotton wadding in the top of the bottle to cushion them.

WORKSHEET 15-2   Cardiac Antidysrhythmics

Name five important components of the conduction system.

a.

b.

c.

d.

e.

Read about lidocaine (Xylocaine). What special preparation must be used if the medication is prescribed to treat dysrhythmia?

Cinchonism is a particular problem with one of the dysrhythmic medications. What is cinchonism? What are the signs and symptoms?

Mrs. Brower comes into the hospital emergency room with a heart rate of 115 and many premature ventricular contractions (PVCs). The doctor orders quinidine for her condition. What is the action of quinidine?

The doctor orders a bolus of lidocaine to be given stat to Mrs. Brower. Why would this be used along with the quinidine?

(Continued)

WORKSHEET 15-2   Cardiac Antidysrhythmics *(cont'd)*

6. Mrs. St. Germaine presents with a very slow, irregular heart rate of 48. Would propranolol (Inderal) be a good drug to increase the heart rate in patients with bradydysrhythmias?

7. Mrs. Dradel comes into the hospital with an atrial tachycardia of 160. Which medication might the physician order for her and why?

8. Mr. Farmer has taken propranolol for the last 4 months for sinus tachycardia. He complains of weight gain, shortness of breath, and dizziness. What is the probable cause of these symptoms?

9. Mr. Billings comes into the hospital with a very irregular pulse. He reports that he has been feeling lightheaded, dizzy, and a little nauseated. He loses consciousness in the emergency room. An ECG shows runs of premature ventricular contractions. What medication is likely to be given first and why?

10. Mr. Richards comes into the clinic for his monthly visit. He is taking digoxin, disopyramide, and hydrochlorothiazide. On this visit he complains of not feeling well, noting especially fatigue, a very dry mouth, constipation, and some urinary retention. The most likely cause of his symptoms is:

WORKSHEET 15-3   Antihyperlipidemics

1. Lipoproteins are
   1. present in the bloodstream, circulating freely as fat globules.
   2. composed of different proportions of high-density and low-density lipids.
   3. also called *chylomicrons* and are formed during absorption of dietary fat in the intestine.
   4. synthesized by the liver and distributed by the blood to tissues throughout the body.
2. The four types of lipoprotein complexes are
   1. chylomicrons, very low-density lipoproteins, ultralow-density lipoproteins, prothrombin protein, low-density lipoproteins.
   2. very low-density lipoproteins, ultralow-density lipoproteins, low-density lipoproteins, very high-density lipoproteins.
   3. chylomicrons, very low-density lipoproteins, low-density lipoproteins, high-density lipoproteins.
   4. cholestyramine, type 1 lipoproteins, very low-density lipoproteins, very high-density lipoproteins.
3. Hyperlipidemia refers to
   1. abnormal lipoprotein patterns in the blood.
   2. atherosclerosis.
   3. occlusive arterial disease.
   4. problems with lipid metabolism.
4. Abnormal elevations of lipids may produce
   1. hypertension.
   2. atherosclerosis.
   3. renal disease.
   4. hepatic failure.
5. Bile acid sequestrants act by
   1. dissolving xanthamatous lipid deposits.
   2. producing excess bile acids to be reabsorbed in the intestine.
   3. inhibiting formation of cholesterol.
   4. forming insoluble complexes with bile salts, increasing bile loss through the feces.
6. Antihyperlipidemic agents such as clofibrate act to
   1. inhibit formation of cholesterol, cause excretion of neutral sterols, and increase breakdown of free fatty acids in the liver.
   2. increase hepatic synthesis of very low-density lipoproteins.
   3. increase binding of free fatty acids to albumin.
   4. increase release of VLDL from the liver to plasma.
7. Bile acid sequestrants are used in the treatment of which of the following problems?
   1. Type I hyperlipidemias
   2. Type II hyperlipidemias
   3. Type III hyperlipidemias
   4. Type IV hyperlipidemias
   5. Type V hyperlipidemias
8. Antihyperlipidemic agents, especially HMG CoA reductase inhibitors, are used in the treatment of which of the following problems?
   1. Type I hyperlipidemias
   2. Type II hyperlipidemias
   3. Type III hyperlipidemias
   4. Type IV hyperlipidemias
   5. Type V hyperlipidemias

(Continued)

WORKSHEET 15-3   Antihyperlipidemics *(cont'd)*

9. Adverse reactions that are produced by medications used in treating lipid disturbances include
    1. constipation, fecal impaction, bizarre dreams.
    2. foul-smelling perspiration, floating stools, frothy urine.
    3. vitamin A deficiency, disturbances in liver function, fecal impaction.
    4. disturbances in liver function, GI upset, diarrhea, constipation.

10. A drug interaction consideration of antihyperlipidemic drugs is that they
    1. interfere with normal absorption of water-soluble vitamins.
    2. are rarely involved in interactions with other drugs.
    3. may produce bleeding problems.
    4. are most effective in very obese patients.

11. Items to stress in teaching patients who are taking these medications include
    1. patients should avoid taking any form of vitamin A supplements, since these may interfere with the drug's efficacy.
    2. use of this medication replaces the need for the patient to be on any special diet.
    3. any other medication ordered by the physician should be taken at the same time as this medication.
    4. notify the doctor if you develop any bleeding or other persistent problems involved with your digestion or bowels.

WORKSHEET 15-4   Antihypertensives

Which of the following is essential to include in the historical evaluation of a patient with known or suspected hypertension?
1. Family history of premature death from stroke or heart attack
2. Current use of oral birth control pills
3. Level of previous blood pressure readings
4. Presence of end organ damage

High blood pressure resulting from a known disease or other problem is called
1. primary hypertension.
2. secondary hypertension.
3. hypercholesteremia.
4. postural hypotension.

Systolic blood pressure is a reflection of
1. the ability of the heart to pump through the circulatory system.
2. cardiac output measured in mm Hg.
3. the highest amount of pressure in the arterial system in mm Hg.
4. the lowest amount of pressure in the arterial system in mm Hg.

Diastolic blood pressure is a reflection of
1. the ability of the heart to pump through the circulatory system.
2. cardiac output measured in mm Hg.
3. the highest amount of pressure in the arterial system in mm Hg.
4. the lowest amount of pressure in the arterial system measured in mm Hg.

A blood pressure of 150/114 would be classified as
1. mild hypertension.
2. moderate hypertension.
3. severe hypertension.
4. malignant hypertension.

Treatment of the hypertensive patient should begin
1. after he has evidence of vascular disease.
2. after the age of 50, regardless of associated disease.
3. as soon as hypertension is detected.
4. if his diastolic pressure is over 120 mm Hg.

Diuretics are used in hypertension to
1. promote fluid loss from the body.
2. encourage reabsorption of sodium and chloride in the thick, ascending loop of Henle and in both proximal and distal kidney tubules.
3. flush toxic metabolites, which are causing hypertension, from the circulatory system.
4. promote weight loss in more obese hypertensive patients.

Adrenergic inhibitors reduce blood pressure through
1. acceleration of cardiac impulses that increase the force of cardiac contraction of the heart.
2. the plugging of alpha and beta receptor sites so that epinephrine and norepinephrine neurotransmitters cannot make contact with the cardiac receptors, preventing cardiac stimulation.
3. nonselective blockage of renin release, which increases the flow of sympathetic vasoconstrictor and cardioaccelerator messages from the brain stem to the vasomotor center.
4. stimulation of sympathetic outflow from the brain, leading to vascular relaxation and lower blood pressure.

(Continued)

WORKSHEET 15-4   Antihypertensives *(cont'd)*

9. Interference in the conversion of specific enzymes from the liver and lungs that plays a role in increased blood pressure is caused by
    1. angiotensin-converting enzyme inhibitor.
    2. aldosterone.
    3. juxtaglomerular apparatus complex.
    4. alpha-adrenergic inhibitors.

10. Vasodilators reduce both systolic and diastolic blood pressure through
    1. competition with alpha-adrenergic receptor sites.
    2. increasing peripheral resistance.
    3. increased diuresis.
    4. direct relaxation of vascular smooth muscle.

11. Slow channel calcium entry blocking agents work through
    1. ion transfer for direct relaxation of vascular smooth muscle.
    2. selective passage of extracellular calcium ions, which promotes increased diuresis.
    3. increased permeability of cardiac membrane.
    4. inhibited passage of extracellular calcium ions through cardiac cell membrane, producing decreased peripheral vascular resistance.

WORKSHEET 15-5   Stepped-Care Regimen in Antihypertensive Therapy

1. The stepped-care treatment regimen for antihypertensive medications begins with the use of
   1. lifestyle modifications.
   2. an adrenergic-inhibiting agent or a loop diuretic in younger patients.
   3. guanethidine in adults or a vasodilator in some younger patients.
   4. a vasodilator in adults or an ACE inhibitor in some younger patients.

2. The third level of antihypertensive treatment is started when
   1. maximal doses of thiazide diuretic fail to lower the blood pressure to the desired level.
   2. antiadrenergic agents have been ineffective.
   3. the patient cannot tolerate step-two drugs.
   4. the patient has adverse reactions to step-two drugs.

3. An example of a step-three drug is
   1. guanethidine.
   2. hydrochlorothiazide.
   3. furosemide.
   4. hydralazine.

4. Step-three drugs are commonly associated with the potentially serious side effect of
   1. depression.
   2. increased risk of breast cancer.
   3. orthostatic hypotension.
   4. impotence.

5. Thiazide therapy is frequently associated with adverse reactions such as
   1. hyperkalemia, hyperuricemia, glucose intolerance.
   2. hypokalemia, hyperuricemia, glucose intolerance, impotence.
   3. hyperkalemia, severe postural hypotension, diabetes.
   4. depression, bizarre dreams.

6. Beta-adrenergic blockers are associated with adverse reactions such as
   1. bradycardia, insomnia, fatigue, bizarre dreams.
   2. tachycardia, asthma, wakefulness, weakness.
   3. sexual dysfunction.
   4. first-dose syncope.

7. A medication often producing positive ANA blood tests is
   1. minoxidil.
   2. hydralazine.
   3. prazosin.
   4. hydrochlorothiazide.

8. First-dose syncope is associated with
   1. guanethidine.
   2. reserpine.
   3. prazosin.
   4. hydrochlorothiazide.

WORKSHEET 15-6   Antihypertensive Therapy

1. Mr. Green has been taking furosemide 100 mg daily for the last 7 months. His blood pressure today is 156/98. Which of the following assessments would be important to report to the physician?
   1. A 10-pound weight gain this week and edema of the feet
   2. Depression
   3. A feeling of weakness when he is walking and climbing
   4. Itching of the hands and scalp

2. Ms. Wright has been taking hydrochlorothiazide 50 mg/day. Her blood pressure today is 140/102. The physician may
   1. stop the hydrochlorothiazide.
   2. increase the hydrochlorothiazide.
   3. add methyldopa, propranolol, or pindolol.
   4. begin guanethidine.

3. Ms. Partridge is 48 years old and has a mild blood pressure elevation for which she receives a step-two drug. Lately she reports having very strange dreams that are unusually vivid. The medication she is taking is most likely
   1. minoxidil.
   2. propranolol.
   3. captopril.
   4. tenormin.

4. Mr. Michaels, 76, comes in today for a routine blood pressure check. His blood pressure is 130/60 in the right arm, sitting position. He takes propranolol 20 mg bid. Mr. Michaels had a myocardial infarction last year but has been without pain since that time. Today he complains of dizziness, shortness of breath, and a slow pulse. These findings may suggest that Mr. Michaels
   1. is having another myocardial infarction.
   2. is having a dosage-related reaction to propranolol.
   3. needs to have his medication increased.
   4. is just getting old and this is to be expected.

5. Ms. Ellis is to begin taking prazosin for her blood pressure, which is currently 178/96. What would you tell her about taking this medication?
   1. The drug may cause excessive drowsiness, which will pass after 2 weeks.
   2. She must take the medication while in the office or hospital and remain there in order that her reaction to the medication be evaluated. Some people pass out after taking the first dose of this medication.
   3. She must drink orange juice and eat potassium-rich foods with this drug.
   4. This drug may cause unusual hair growth.

WORKSHEET 15-7   Cardiotonic Medications

1. One of the most important effects of digitalis is its positive inotropic action. This effect is shown when
   1. the heart rate is increased.
   2. the strength of each heart contraction is increased.
   3. cardiac output decreases.
   4. mechanical energy is converted into chemical energy.

2. Digitalization is the process of bringing the patient's decompensated or irregularly beating heart under control. This is usually accomplished by giving
   1. one very large dose of digitalis.
   2. only the amount of digitalis that will produce the desired effects.
   3. a small dose of digitalis daily.
   4. a small dose of digitalis on admission to the hospital.

3. Individuals may gradually retain large amounts of digitalis in the body and develop signs and symptoms of digitalis toxicity. Signs to look for include
   1. anorexia, nausea, weakness, drowsiness, visual changes.
   2. diarrhea, cardiac dysrhythmias, excessive fatigue, productive cough.
   3. rapid weight gain, shortness of breath, productive cough.
   4. edema of the hands and feet, headaches, chest pain.

4. Which of the factors listed here is likely to be associated with a high risk of developing digitalis toxicity?
   1. CNS problems
   2. Administration of diuretics
   3. Administration of electrolytes
   4. Rapid digitalization

5. In the event of potassium loss (such as when a patient is receiving concurrent diuretic therapy), it may be necessary to increase the dietary intake of potassium-rich foods. These include
   1. green leafy vegetables.
   2. fish.
   3. fresh fruits.
   4. bananas and citrus fruits.

6. Before administering an ordered dose of a digitalis medication, the nurse should
   1. check the medication label for the name of the drug, because names of various drugs are sometimes similar and can be easily confused.
   2. check the accuracy of the dosage.
   3. take the patient's pulse before giving the medication.
   4. take the patient's blood pressure before giving the medication.

7. The nurse should observe the client receiving digitalis for signs of improvement. Signs of positive response would include
   1. an increase in edema, including the size of the fluid-swollen abdomen and pitting edema in the ankles, tibia, and sacral region.
   2. an increase in daily urinary output and a decrease in daily weight.
   3. an increase in signs and symptoms of pulmonary congestion.
   4. a gradual increase of the pulse to between 70 and 80 beats per minute.

(Continued)

WORKSHEET 15-7   Cardiotonic Medications *(cont'd)*

8. Mr. Doxey is receiving a digitalis preparation. You are assessing his condition to determine whether the drug therapy is working. You observe that his edema has decreased, his urinary output has increased, his weight has dropped, his pulmonary congestion has decreased, and his pulse rate is 80 beats per minute. You can infer that
    1. chronic heart failure is still present.
    2. there is still evidence of renal impairment.
    3. digitalis therapy has been helpful.
    4. the underlying dysrhythmia is unchanged.

9. Mrs. Black, age 68, has been hospitalized for treatment of chronic heart failure and is now returning home. She is receiving oral digitoxin and will be administering the medication herself. Which of the following instructions will you provide to Mrs. Black?
    1. Explain the action, purpose, and dosage of the medication, as well as the importance of taking it as ordered. She should take the medication after meals.
    2. Explain adverse reactions that may occur and tell her to report them immediately to the physician.
    3. Instruct her about how to take a pulse, recognize abnormal changes in heart rate or rhythm, weigh herself, and keep records of her findings.
    4. Instruct her about diet and provide nutritional guidelines that include foods high in sodium content.

WORKSHEET 15-8   Electrolytes

1. Electrolytes are _____ .

2. The principal intracellular cation of most body tissues that participates in the maintenance of normal renal function, contraction of muscle, and transmission of nerve impulses is _____ .

3. Nausea, vomiting, diarrhea, abdominal discomfort, along with flaccid paralysis, mental confusion, restlessness, weakness, and heaviness of the legs may suggest _____ or _____ .

4. Potassium comes in various salt combinations. The form most frequently prescribed is _____ .

5. Symptoms of dehydration might include _____ .

6. Fluids and electrolytes may be given either orally or parenterally in the following conditions:

   _____ .

◆ Chapter 15—Integrated Case Study ◆

A 50-year-old African American man comes to the clinic with a 1-week history of occipital headache that he describes as "a constant ache in the back of my head." The 650-mg Tylenol that he has taken regularly four to five times daily over the past week often has not cured his headache. Approximately 7 months ago, the patient was told that his blood pressure was "up" during a yearly employment physical. He has a history of asthma, gout, and angina. His father and sister have high blood pressure. His diet is high in fat and salt.

Physical examination: Blood pressure: right arm sitting, 160/105 mm Hg; left arm sitting, 162/104 mm Hg. The heart is not enlarged; there are no murmurs or abnormal rhythms. Apical pulse, 84 beats/minute.

1. Assuming the patient's blood pressure remained at the same level after two subsequent blood pressure checks, what factors, specific to this patient, should be considered before placing the patient on antihypertensive medications?

2. What class of medication would most likely be of greatest help in controlling this patient's blood pressure with the fewest adverse reactions?
    1. Thiazide or loop diuretic
    2. Beta blocker
    3. Alpha blocker
    4. Centrally acting agent
    5. Adrenergic neuron blocking agent
    6. Direct-acting vasodilating agent
    7. Angiotensin-converting enzyme inhibitor
    8. Calcium channel blocker

3. Which of the drugs listed in question 2 would not be indicated?

4. The doctor orders hydrochlorothiazide 12.5 mg daily. What would you tell the patient about this drug?

5. Assuming the drug was ineffective in reducing the patient's blood pressure after 4 weeks, what could be done to achieve adequate control of the blood pressure?

Central and Peripheral Nervous System Medications

Answer Key: A complete answer key was provided for your instructor.

OBJECTIVES

1. Identify the major classes of drugs that affect the central nervous system.
2. Explain the major actions of drugs used to treat disorders of the central nervous system.
3. List different actions of antimigraine products.
4. Identify the role of psychotropic drugs in psychotherapeutic intervention.
5. Compare and contrast different categories of medications used to treat depression.

Be sure to check out the bonus material on the free CD-ROM in your textbook, including:

Audio Pronunciation Guide
NCLEX®-Style Review Questions: Chapter 16
Top 200 Drugs by Prescription

WORKSHEET 16-1   Antimigraine Medications: Thought Questions

1. Explain the physiologic mechanism that produces migraine headaches.

2. How do antimigraine products act to reduce pain from migraine headaches?

3. What is the oxytocic effect of adrenergic-blocking agents?

4. Why may chronic overdosage of antimigraine medications easily occur?

5. What effect does the use of migraine agents at the onset of an attack have on the efficacy of these drugs in relieving migraine pain and symptoms?

6. What is added to the antimigraine product to speed up absorption of oral and rectal preparations?

7. Abrupt discontinuation of migraine agents after prolonged use can result in
   1. withdrawal symptoms.
   2. strokes.
   3. damage to the uterus.
   4. rebound headaches.

8. The medication used in prophylaxis of migraine headaches is _____.

9. Some antimigraine products contain other chemicals. List three other ingredients and explain why they are included.

WORKSHEET 16-2   Anticonvulsants

1. What is the physiologic mechanism that produces the symptoms of epilepsy?

2. List the four major groups of drugs used to treat seizures.

3. Barbiturates that are _____ acting make up the primary category of anticonvulsants used to treat _____ seizures and are used for their _____ effect on the brain.

4. Name two adverse reactions to barbiturates.

5. A risk of long-term use of barbiturates is _____ .

6. Explain why elderly patients may require smaller doses of barbiturates than other patients.

7. Barbiturates are classed as both anticonvulsants and sedatives. Why are they controlled substances?

8. What may be the effect of administering barbiturates to steroid-dependent asthmatics?

9. Are barbiturates given adjunctively to help control pain?

(Continued)

WORKSHEET 16-2   Anticonvulsants *(cont'd)*

10. Name the benzodiazepines used to treat seizures.

11. Identify the benzodiazepine that is the drug of choice in treating status epilepticus.

12. The other two benzodiazepines are used in the treatment of _____ seizures.

13. How are benzodiazepines changed in the liver? Although the drugs are helpful in controlling seizures, why might they become a problem for the patient?

14. Hydantoins are commonly used for the treatment of _____ .

15. Adverse reactions to hydantoins are common. List them.

16. Benzodiazepines are noted for their lack of drug interactions. Name some of the most important potential interactions with other drugs.

17. Name a group of anticonvulsants that interferes with the accuracy of some laboratory tests.

18. Hydantoin comes in either **prompt** or **extended** capsules. Which do you think would be better for a patient beginning hydantoin therapy?

    Why?

(Continued)

WORKSHEET 16-2   Anticonvulsants *(cont'd)*

19. The doctor writes a prescription for a specific brand of hydantoin and asks the pharmacist not to change it. Why would this be done?

20. Succinimides are used primarily in the treatment of _____ seizures.

21. Identify the adverse reactions of succinimides.

22. Name three miscellaneous medications used in anticonvulsant therapy.

23. Compare the various types of anticonvulsant medications, and list the ways in which all the groups are similar.

24. Compare the various types of anticonvulsant medications and list ways in which the groups differ.

WORKSHEET 16-3   Antiemetic and Antivertigo Drugs

1. List three physiologic mechanisms that produce nausea or vomiting.

    a.

    b.

    c.

2. Identify four common causes of nausea or vomiting.

    a.

    b.

    c.

    d.

3. List four anticholinergic medications used to control motion sickness.

    a.

    b.

    c.

    d.

4. List three medications used to control vertigo.

    a.

    b.

    c.

5. The most common side effect of antihistamines is:

6. Anticholinergic medications produce other side effects such as:

(Continued)

WORKSHEET 16-3   Antiemetic and Antivertigo Drugs *(cont'd)*

7. Pregnancy is a common cause of nausea. Which medications should be used to control symptoms of morning sickness?

8. These medications come in several forms. When might sustained action capsules, suppositories, or injections be indicated?

9. If medications are given to prevent motion sickness, when should the patient be told to take the medication?

10. What common special precaution should be given to all patients taking these medications?

11. Scopolamine comes in a unique dosage form. What is this form and what general information should you give the patient about it?

12. Your patient is placed on a phenothiazine derivative. What changes in the urine might be produced by this medication?

WORKSHEET 16-4   Antiparkinsonian Agents

1. Describe the basic disorder in Parkinson's disease, and list some of the signs and symptoms observed in the patient with Parkinson's disease.

2. Identify the two main pharmacologic actions of antiparkinsonian agents.

    a.

    b.

3. What is the therapeutic response desired in treatment of Parkinson's disease?

4. The two major categories of drugs used to treat Parkinson's disease are _____ and _____ drugs.

5. Compare the actions of amantadine, bromocriptine, and levodopa.

6. List at least five common side effects of the two common categories of medications used to treat Parkinson's disease.

7. What are the early signs of toxicity in the patient taking dopaminergic agents?

(Continued)

WORKSHEET 16-4   Antiparkinsonian Agents *(cont'd)*

8. What is blepharospasm? (Consult a medical dictionary.)

9. What are the symptoms of overdosage with these medications?

10. Circle the correct answer: Dopaminergic agents interact with (relatively few, very many) drugs.

11. Using a medical dictionary when necessary, define the following terms.

Akinesia

Tardive dyskinesia

Dystonia

Cogwheel rigidity of limbs

Athetosis

Chorea

Bradykinesia

Tics

12. List at least three anticholinergic medications.

13. List at least three dopaminergic agents.

14. What special precautions should be given to a patient with Parkinson's disease who is taking anticholinergic medications during the summer?

WORKSHEET 16-5   Antianxiety Agents

1. Anxiety is a (subjective, objective) finding, producing feelings of _____
    _____.

    The nurse may also observe _____.

2. Why should antianxiety agents be given for only a short period of time?

3. What is a major risk with antianxiety agents that are given for a long period of time?

4. Identify the major category of medications used to treat anxiety.

5. Name several benzodiazepine drug interactions.

6. Benzodiazepines may cause gastrointestinal distress. What might you teach the patient about avoiding or
    decreasing this problem?

7. Why are benzodiazepines controlled substances?

8. Which age groups would have the greatest potential for problems in taking benzodiazepines?

    _____

    Why?

9. What are common contraindications to benzodiazepines?

WORKSHEET 16-6   Antidepressant Medications

1. Name the three major categories of medications used to treat depression.

2. Name three antidepressants that are not from the categories listed in question 1.

3. What is the probable mechanism of action for the tricyclic antidepressants?

4. Why have tricyclic antidepressants replaced MAO inhibitors as the usual drugs of choice?

5. What general patterns are seen with drug overdosage of tricyclic antidepressants?

6. Why are tricyclic antidepressants and MAO inhibitors not usually used conjunctively?

7. What is the probable mechanism of action of MAO inhibitors?

8. What is the general pattern of overdosage with MAO inhibitors?

9. What instructions would you give patients regarding their diets or prn medication use while they are taking MAO inhibitors?

(Continued)

WORKSHEET 16-6   Antidepressant Medications *(cont'd)*

10. What is the specific chemical in food that interacts with MAO inhibitors?

11. List at least five foods that would be contraindicated for patients receiving MAO inhibitors.

12. Why are these foods avoided?

13. Identify one thing antidepressant medications that do not fall into the three major categories have in common regarding their use.

14. Bupropion HCl has been noted for producing what adverse reaction?

15. What is the recommended drug dosage for fluoxetine?

16. What is the unique action of trazodone compared to other antidepressants?

17. Identify an important thing to stress when teaching the family or patient about bupropion HCl, fluoxetine, or trazodone.

18. Compare the antidepressant medications. Which group of medications presents the most risk of adverse reactions to the patient?

WORKSHEET 16-7   Antipsychotic Medications

1. The three categories of medications used in treating psychotic patients include the _____ and _____ and the _____.

2. Most antipsychotic agents work by _____.

3. If different antipsychotic agents use the same mechanism, how do they differ?

4. Antipsychotic agents produce side effects on different body systems. Give examples that support this statement.

5. In addition to their antipsychotic action, phenothiazines may also be used for _____ and _____.

6. When are thioxanthene derivatives preferable to phenothiazines?

7. Identify the symptoms of phenothiazine overdosage.

8. Name at least three potentially serious adverse reactions of the phenothiazines.

9. Why should the patient avoid activities that cause excessive sweating and urination?

10. Name the three nonphenothiazine antipsychotics.

(Continued)

WORKSHEET 16-7   Antipsychotic Medications *(cont'd)*

11. Loxapine is chemically similar to which other group of antipsychotic medications?

12. What drug interactions should you look for with molindone?

13. Why should families or patient support systems be involved in the teaching plans for antipsychotics?

WORKSHEET 16-8   Antimanics

1. Why is lithium unique when compared to all other psychiatric drugs?

2. Lithium is used for the _____ and _____ of
    acute _____.

3. List at least four adverse reactions of lithium.

4. Identify the symptoms of lithium overdosage.

5. Toxicity may easily be produced by concurrent use of _____.

6. What problem develops when the therapeutic range and the toxic range of a medication are close together?

7. In monitoring lithium blood levels, when should the blood specimen be drawn?

WORKSHEET 16-9   Sedative-Hypnotics

1. What is meant by "sedative"?

2. What is meant by "hypnotic"?

3. How could a medication used as a sedative also be a hypnotic?

4. What are the four stages of sleep?

5. What is REM and when does it occur?

6. What are common classifications of insomnia?

7. What are nonpharmacologic approaches the patient may take to try to resolve insomnia?

(Continued)

WORKSHEET 16-9   Sedative-Hypnotics *(cont'd)*

8. Why do patients feel lethargic or "hung over" after taking a sedative medication?

9. What is a common physiologic mechanism leading to psychologic dependence on these medications?

10. Three different groups of medications have sedative-hypnotic effects. Name them.

11. The safest group of medications to use for sedation-hypnosis is the _____.

12. Develop a specific teaching plan for a patient who is going home from the hospital and will be taking one of these medications to help relieve general tension and anxiety.

13. Legally, these medications are considered _____ substances. What does that mean regarding nursing responsibility in administering these medications while the patient is in the hospital?

14. You receive a phone call from a patient who has gone home from the hospital saying that he has had a difficult time sleeping, does not feel refreshed, and has long and vivid dreams. What would you tell the patient?

◆ Chapter 16—Integrated Case Study ◆

Mrs. Jane Michner, a 65-year-old widow, was admitted 2 weeks ago with a fractured hip. She has a 6-year history of Parkinson's disease. Her hip is healing well, but she is having difficulty learning to walk with crutches. This has made her very depressed, and she is concerned about how she will manage when she returns home. She has also developed symptoms of a urinary tract infection, a problem she has had repeatedly. She is currently receiving:

    Ascorbic acid (vitamin C): 1 gm PO 4 times daily
    Levodopa (Larodopa): 1 gm PO 3 times daily with meals
    Nitrofurantoin (Macrodantin): 100 mg PO 3 times daily

1.   Why is Mrs. Michner taking ascorbic acid?

2.   What special information do you need to give Mrs. Michner about her antiparkinsonian medications?

3.   Several days after admission, Mrs. Michner developed a maculopapular eruption of the skin all over her trunk. What is the likely cause of this problem?

4.   What medications might Mrs. Michner take to treat the urinary tract infection?

5.   The doctor starts Mrs. Michner on imipramine HCl (Tofranil) 20 mg PO twice daily. Why was this drug ordered? What does the patient need to know about it?

6.   Does Mrs. Michner have any contraindications to the use of imipramine HCl?

17 Medications for Pain Management

Answer Key: A complete answer key was provided for your instructor.

OBJECTIVES

List medications commonly used for the treatment of moderate to severe pain.
Evaluate different forms of narcotic agonists and narcotic agonist-antagonists in their ability to control pain.
Explain why there are so many rules about how narcotics and related analgesic drugs may be given.
Compare and contrast drug tolerance and drug addiction.
List behavior that would make you believe a patient is addicted to the drug.

Be sure to check out the bonus material on the free CD-ROM in your textbook, including:

Audio Pronunciation Guide
NCLEX®-Style Review Questions: Chapter 17
Top 200 Drugs by Prescription

WORKSHEET 17-1   Narcotics

True/False

Narcotic agonist analgesics are used to treat _____.

1. T   F   The acute pain of myocardial infarction
2. T   F   A persistent cough
3. T   F   The pain associated with labor and delivery
4. T   F   Dyspnea related to left ventricular failure
5. T   F   Postoperative pain
6   T   F   Acute renal colic
7. T   F   Detoxification of narcotic addiction

8. Why are narcotics used primarily in the hospital rather than in outpatient settings?

9. Narcotics have been associated with many adverse reactions. Name a few of the most frequently seen reactions.

10. Overdosage with narcotics may be either chronic or acute. Give the symptoms to monitor for each type of overdosage.

    Acute:

    Chronic:

11. Based on your answers in questions 3 and 4, construct a teaching plan for a patient and family about narcotic therapy.

12. The CNS depressant effects of narcotic analgesics may be increased by coadministration with:

(Continued)

WORKSHEET 17-1   Narcotics *(cont'd)*

13. Which of the following behaviors might be considered signs of dependence?
    1. Asking for pain medication every 3 to 4 hours postoperatively for 2 to 3 days.
    2. Requesting an increased dosage and frequency of medication administration.
    3. Receiving care for a problem from several different physicians or agencies.
    4. A history of dependence or abuse.
    5. A clinical problem that produces chronic pain.
    6. Inability to wean from the drug.

14. How does a narcotic agonist-antagonist differ from a narcotic agonist?

15. Why might a narcotic agonist-antagonist be preferred to a narcotic agonist for outpatient ambulatory use?

16. Name the three drugs that make up the narcotic agonist-antagonist category.

17. List the most common adverse reactions and overdosage symptoms of the narcotic agonist-antagonist medications.

18. What are the most common narcotics found in narcotic-combination products?

19. What are the major nonnarcotic ingredients in narcotic analgesic combination products?

20. Mr. Sykes is an inpatient recovering from surgery following a ruptured appendix. He had a severe postoperative infection with high temperatures and excessive pain. He has been receiving codeine 32 mg prn, Amoxil 500 mg qid, and Tylenol 650 mg q4h for the last 4 days. He is complaining of constipation. What has caused the constipation? What would you recommend for the patient to relieve the constipation?

WORKSHEET 17-2   Nonnarcotic Analgesics

1. Identify at least three groups of nonnarcotics used for analgesia.

Multiple Choice

2. These medications are generally used for relief of
    1. mild pain.
    2. moderate pain.
    3. severe pain.

3. These medications cause many minor side effects. The most common adverse reactions include
    1. orthostatic hypotension, dizziness, sedation, nausea, and vomiting.
    2. disorientation, headache, and lightheadedness.
    3. cyanosis and slurring of speech.
    4. blood dyscrasias, epigastric distress, and chills.

4. Examine the drug interactions listed for this group of drugs and compare them with the drug interactions for the narcotic agonist and narcotic agonist-antagonist groups. Do you see any similarities?

5. _____ is a medication characterized by a high incidence of orthostatic hypotension, fainting, dizziness, or sedation, especially during the first 6 hours of use.

6. Specific assessments to make on the patient receiving these medications include:

Chapter 17—Integrated Case Study ◆

Mr. Rim, a hard-working Korean immigrant, works in an inner-city convenience store. He has recently hurt his back lifting heavy boxes.

What would be the most appropriate form of initial pain control?

The pain continues and now Mr. Rim experiences pain shooting from his lower back down his left leg. X-ray studies reveal a ruptured vertebral disk and he undergoes surgery. What type of analgesia is likely to be ordered after surgery?

Mr. Rim does not want to take any pain medication. He believes that he should only have pain medication if his pain is so bad that he cannot tolerate it. What would you tell him?

Is there any reason why Mr. Rim is likely to become addicted to this medicine because of his ethnic background?

What type of behavior might lead you to believe that a patient has become addicted to pain medicine?

Gastrointestinal Medications

Answer Key: A complete answer key was provided for your instructor.

OBJECTIVES

1. Identify common uses for antacids and histamine H_2-receptor antagonists.
2. Compare and contrast the actions of anticholinergic and antispasmodic medications on the gastrointestinal (GI) tract.
3. Compare the actions and adverse reactions of the five major classifications of laxatives.
4. Identify indications for the use of at least two common antidiarrheals, antiflatulents, digestive enzymes, and emetics.
5. Describe indications for disulfiram use and what is meant by "disulfiram reaction."

⏺ **Be sure to check out the bonus material on the free CD-ROM in your textbook, including:**

Audio Pronunciation Guide
NCLEX®-Style Review Questions: Chapter 18
Top 200 Drugs by Prescription

WORKSHEET 18-1   Antacids and Histamine H₂-Receptor Antagonists

Indicate the actions of antacids and histamine H$_2$-receptor antagonists by putting an "**A**" (antacids); "**H**" (histamine H$_2$-receptor antagonists); "**B**" (both); or "**N**" (neither) in front of the following possible actions.

1. _____   Neutralize hydrochloric acid

2. _____   Increase gastric pH

3. _____   Increase hydrogen ion absorption

4. _____   Buffer gastric acid

5. _____   Inhibit secretion of gastric acid

6. _____   Tighten gastric mucosa

7. _____   Decrease gastric pH

8. _____   Promote healing of gastric and duodenal ulcers

9. _____   Increase tone of cardiac sphincter

10. _____   Formation of gas

1. How may antacids can be associated with hypermagnesemia?

2. If a patient is taking an anticoagulant, which H$_2$ histamine blocker is the medication least likely to interfere with the anticoagulant?

3. Why should a person taking cimetidine not smoke?

4. How can patients avoid problems with diarrhea or constipation from antacid use?

WORKSHEET 18-2   Anticholinergics, Antispasmodics, Antidiarrheals

1. Name at least five adverse reactions seen with anticholinergics.

2. Antispasmodic effects are basically (the same as, different from) anticholinergic effects.

3. Antidiarrheal agents (do, do not) act in the same manner as anticholinergic agents.

4. Mr. Frank, age 84, comes in to the clinic with mild abdominal discomfort, increased flatus, and watery stools. His history is negative except for mild prostatic hypertrophy. Mr. Frank (would, would not) be a good candidate for anticholinergic therapy. Why or why not?

5. Because Mr. Frank is elderly and has had prolonged diarrhea, what particular problems must the nurse anticipate?

6. Would there be any contraindication to starting Mr. Frank on Lomotil?

7. Mr. Frank said that he had been restricting fluid intake so that he did not have so much diarrhea. What would you tell him?

(Continued)

WORKSHEET 18-2   Anticholinergics, Antispasmodics, Antidiarrheals *(cont'd)*

8. Long-term anticholinergic therapy may mask or alter symptoms of gastrointestinal disease. Why might this be a problem?

9. Dietary modifications are usually a part of the treatment regimen for any GI disease. What sort of modifications might be anticipated?

10. Some antidiarrheal medications may contain habit-forming substances. How does that influence their use?

WORKSHEET 18-3   Laxatives

Fill in the following chart.

	Type of Laxative	Action	Uses
1.			
2.			
3.			
4.			
5.			

6. Identify the common side effects of laxatives.

7. List at least four ideas important in teaching a patient about laxative use.

8. Why might laxatives that contain sodium be contraindicated in a patient with chronic heart failure?

◆ Chapter 18—Integrated Case Study ◆

Mr. Frost is a 73-year-old man who is being treated for CHF that developed after an acute myocardial infarction. His stay in the hospital has been upsetting for him, and both his eating and bowel habits have changed. He usually reports a bowel movement every morning but has been unable to pass stool for the last 3 days. He is currently sitting on a commode and straining. The doctor orders:

Metamucil: 1 rounded tsp 1 to 2 times/day
Lanoxin: 0.25 mg PO daily
Hydrochlorothiazide: 50 mg daily

1. Why is the Metamucil ordered?

2. If the Metamucil does not work, what type of laxative might be effective?

3. What type of laxative would not be indicated for this patient?

4. Why is the Lanoxin ordered?

5. What is the purpose of the hydrochlorothiazide?

6. Are there any things to be concerned about in a patient taking hydrochlorothiazide?

7. What dietary modifications might assist Mr. Frost in returning to normal bowel activity?

Hematologic Products

Answer Key: A complete answer key was provided for your instructor.

OBJECTIVES

1. Identify drugs that act in the formation, repair, or function of red blood cells.
2. Describe the influence of anticoagulants on blood clotting.
3. Identify at least three adverse reactions associated with hematologic products.
4. Develop a teaching plan for patients taking anticoagulants on a long-term basis.

⊙ **Be sure to check out the bonus material on the free CD-ROM in your textbook, including:**

Audio Pronunciation Guide
NCLEX®-Style Review Questions: Chapter 19
Top 200 Drugs by Prescription

WORKSHEET 19-1   Anticoagulants

1. A clot formed from fibrin, platelets, and cholesterol that either attaches to the inner wall of a blood vessel or occupies the entire lumen of a vessel is called
   1. a thrombus.
   2. an embolism.

2. A blood clot that becomes detached from thrombophlebitis in the lower extremities and is free to travel through the circulation is called
   1. a thrombus.
   2. an embolism.

3. Which of the following reflects heparin's mechanism of action?
   1. It interferes with the metabolic functions of vitamin K and hinders the biochemical reactions that result in the liver's synthesis of prothrombin and coagulation factors VII, IX, and X.
   2. It interferes with the formation of thrombin and increases the action of antithrombin III on several other coagulation factors, primarily factor Xa.

4. In order to maintain a constant level of heparin in the blood, it should be administered in which of the following ways?
   1. Orally
   2. Subcutaneously
   3. Intermittent IV infusion
   4. Continuous IV infusion

5. Intravenous injections of heparin are primarily used to
   1. prevent the formation of blood clots or to prevent complete occlusion of blood vessels.
   2. dissolve clots that have already formed in the blood vessels.
   3. reduce the number of clots formed.

6. The most commonly used laboratory test to monitor the effectiveness of heparin is
   1. prothrombin time.
   2. Lee-White clotting time.
   3. partial thrombin time.
   4. activated partial thromboplastin time.

7. Oral coumarin therapy is prescribed when
   1. the patient is not responsive to heparin therapy.
   2. the blood clots need to be dissolved.
   3. long-term anticoagulant therapy is warranted.

8. Coumarin acts by
   1. interfering with the metabolic function of vitamin K and hindering the biochemical reactions that result in the liver's synthesis of prothrombin and coagulation factors VII, IX, and X.
   2. increasing the effectiveness of heparin sodium.
   3. interfering with the formation of thrombin, limiting platelet aggregation.

9. The laboratory test that monitors the effectiveness of coumarin is
   1. Lee-White clotting time.
   2. prothrombin time.
   3. partial thrombin time.

(Continued)

WORKSHEET 19-1   Anticoagulants *(cont'd)*

In questions 10 through 12, indicate whether you believe the patient should be started on anticoagulant therapy.

10. Mr. Ransom is in a nursing home. He is 72 years old, suffering from Alzheimer's disease, and showing marked confusion. He develops acute thrombophlebitis in his left leg. There are no signs of abnormal bleeding or other conditions that would prevent anticoagulant therapy.
    1. Patient should be started on anticoagulant therapy.
    2. Patient should not be started on anticoagulant therapy.

11. Ms. Watson has an acute peptic ulcer and chronic recurrent arterial occlusion.
    1. She should be started on coumarin therapy, but not heparin.
    2. She should be started on heparin therapy, but not coumarin.
    3. She should not be started on either heparin or coumarin.

12. Ms. Willis has just delivered a 10-pound baby boy. She now has symptoms of an acute thrombophlebitis.
    1. She should be started on heparin immediately.
    2. She should not receive heparin.
    3. She should start on coumarin now, if she doesn't breastfeed.

13. When giving a deep subcutaneous (intrafat) injection of heparin the nurse should remember to
    1. pull back gently on the barrel plunger to aspirate very carefully.
    2. massage the area gently after the injection.
    3. consult the rotation chart for the last injection site.

14. Anticoagulants may be given for a variety of reasons. Identify at least one of these reasons.

15. When is heparin the drug of choice?

16. When is coumarin the drug of choice?

17. When is protamine sulfate indicated?

(Continued)

WORKSHEET 19-1   Anticoagulants *(cont'd)*

18. If protamine sulfate is an anticoagulant, why is it used in heparin overdosage?

19. What are common signs of anticoagulant overdosage?

20. What should patients do if they forget to take their oral anticoagulant?

21. How is the dosage of anticoagulant medication determined?

22. When is folic acid indicated?

23. What is a common medication that may produce mild folic acid deficiency?

WORKSHEET 19-2   Thrombolytic and Antiplatelet Agents

1. Thrombolytics convert plasminogen to the enzyme plasmin, which degrades fibrin clots, fibrinogen, and other plasma proteins. Because of this action, when would these products be used?

2. Use of thrombolytics reduces the extent of cellular damage from occlusion. Why?

3. What are possible adverse reactions to thrombolytics?

4. When Mr. Adams visits his doctor for a routine examination and ECG, it is discovered that he has had a silent myocardial infarction (MI) some time within the last few months. Should thrombolytics be started now?

5. What other medications might interfere with thrombolytics?

6. Mrs. Winters is rushed to the hospital with signs of an acute ischemic stroke. She is given a thrombolytic as soon as she arrives in the emergency room. The nurse is told to observe her carefully for bleeding. You note superficial bleeding, coming from the infusion site. Is this significant?

(Continued)

WORKSHEET 19-2   Thrombolytic and Antiplatelet Agents *(cont'd)*

7. How do thrombolytics and antiplatelet agents differ?

8. If a patient is suspected of having a myocardial infarction, what medication can be administered immedi-
    ately?

9. If a patient is admitted with a stroke due to hemorrhage, should aspirin be administered?

10. What three medications are used for MI prophylaxis for men and as adjunct therapy with thrombolytics in
    preventing infarction or stroke?

11. Antiplatelet medications may interact with what medications?

◆ Chapter 19—Integrated Case Study ◆

Mrs. Lily, 34 years old, arrives at the office late for her appointment. She is limping and says her right calf is very sore. It is swollen, red, and very painful to touch. Mrs. Lily is a heavy smoker, takes oral birth control pills, and was recently involved in a car accident in which her right leg was badly bruised. The doctor admits her to the hospital with the following orders:

Bed rest
Right leg elevated and wrapped with warm, moist compresses
Heparin IV q6h

1. If Mrs. Lily has thrombophlebitis, what is the probable cause?

2. What risk factors does she have now for other adverse reactions?

3. What blood test is useful in determining how much heparin should be given?

4. The dosage of heparin is considered adequate when the whole blood clotting time is approximately _____ the control value.

5. Low-intensity coumarin therapy (prothrombin time ratio between 1.2 and 1.5) greatly decreases the risk of stroke from what condition?

6. The doctor also orders Coumadin during Mrs. Lily's stay in the hospital. Why?

7. On admission, Mrs. Lily was found to have a hematocrit of 32% and a hemoglobin of 11 gm/dL. The doctor believes that this is because of blood loss during several pregnancies and heavy periods. What will be the likely course of treatment?

Hormones and Steroids

Answer Key: A complete answer key was provided for your instructor.

OBJECTIVES

1. Describe the use of antidiabetic medications.
2. Identify preparations that act on the uterus.
3. Compare and contrast the action of adrenal and pituitary hormones.
4. Describe at least five adverse reactions that may result from the use of glucocortical and mineralocortical steroids.
5. Compare the actions of various male and female hormones.
6. List the indications for the use of thyroid preparations.

⊙ **Be sure to check out the bonus material on the free CD-ROM in your textbook, including:**

Audio Pronunciation Guide
NCLEX®-Style Review Questions: Chapter 20
Top 200 Drugs by Prescription

WORKSHEET 20-1   Insulin and Oral Antidiabetic Agents

1. If you have a patient who has a diseased, nonfunctioning pancreas, would the patient need insulin or oral antidiabetic medications? The main action of insulin is to stimulate production of more insulin by the beta cells of the pancreas.

2. Insulin helps move glucose into the cells of the body. What would happen if the cells were resistant to the insulin?

3. What role does insulin play in the metabolic processes in the liver affecting fat?

4. If the patient continues to give frequent injections of insulin into the same site, what may be the result?

5. If a diabetic patient begins taking oral contraceptives, what is the influence on the need for insulin?

6. Mrs. Halifax is a brittle diabetic—one with wide variations in blood sugar in response to medications. The nurse must watch her carefully for symptoms of hyperglycemia after giving her an insulin injection. What signs or symptoms is she most concerned about?

(Continued)

WORKSHEET 20-1   Insulin and Oral Antidiabetic Agents *(cont'd)*

7. Identify the symptoms of hypoglycemia.

8. Ted Wiggins is an 18-year-old with type 1 diabetes. He is active in sports and loves to dance. What influence does this type of increase in work or exercise have on his blood sugar level?

9. Mr. John Leavitt is a diabetic with arthritis, coronary artery disease, asthma, and obesity. He works as an aircraft controller at a busy airport. What risk factors does he have for the development of insulin resistance?

10. In counseling Mrs. Wilson, a new diabetic, you discover that she has been administering regular insulin deep IM just before meals. She seems to have confidence in giving the injection and can draw up and read the dosage properly. What suggestions would you give her?

11. In altering Mrs. Wilson's medication the doctor says he will switch her to a longer-acting medication. What is the difference between the onset of action for regular and NPH insulin?

12. The doctor decides to order a combination of regular and NPH insulin for Mrs. Wilson. It is important to tell Mrs. Wilson to
    1. shake the insulin vial well before withdrawing the medication to make certain all chemicals are dissolved.
    2. draw up the regular insulin before drawing up the NPH insulin in the same syringe.
    3. use a different syringe for each injection.

(Continued)

WORKSHEET 20-1   Insulin and Oral Antidiabetic Agents *(cont'd)*

13. What do you think the term *rainbow coverage* might mean for diabetic therapy?
    1. The medication may be given to people of all races and backgrounds.
    2. Different doses of insulin are ordered based on the blood glucose level.
    3. A combination of products is used in treating the person.

14. Mrs. Wilson is instructed to test her sugar level at home in order to determine how much insulin she is to take. She will do this by using a
    1. glucometer to test urine sugar levels.
    2. glucometer to test blood glucose levels.
    3. glucose thermometer to test blood and urine levels.

15. Somogyi effect occurs when _____.

16. The most common adverse reactions with oral hypoglycemic agents are
    1. GI symptoms.
    2. allergy.
    3. high blood pressure.

17. Benny Parks is a 45-year-old homeless alcoholic. He is well known to the local hospital because of his diabetes. Because he was unable to take insulin while living on the streets, the doctor started him on a sulfonylurea. What would you be concerned about?
    1. The medication requires that it be taken with food and Benny may not be eating.
    2. The patient must eat three regular meals a day while taking this medication.
    3. A disulfiram-like reaction may result in some patients if the patient takes sulfonylureas and drinks alcohol.

18. Miss Eldredge is a 64-year-old retired schoolteacher. She has recently been diagnosed with type 2 diabetes. It is important to tell her that
    1. a patient who has type 2 diabetes will never have to take insulin.
    2. she can avoid taking any medication if she will eliminate all carbohydrates from her diet.
    3. medication and diet are both important parts of the treatment plan.

19. The major difference in the oral hypoglycemic agents is in the _____.

20. Sulfonylureas may be associated with
    1. allergies.
    2. thyroid immunodeficiencies.
    3. hepatitis.

WORKSHEET 20-2   Drugs Acting on the Uterus

1. Mrs. Ott comes into the hospital in labor. She is 6 weeks premature. The doctor will most likely order
   1. an abortifacient.
   2. a uterine relaxant.
   3. a muscle relaxant.
   4. an oxytocic or ergot preparation.

2. Following delivery of a baby and placenta, the uterus must clamp down to control bleeding. A medication that might help limit uterine bleeding would be
   1. an abortifacient.
   2. a uterine relaxant.
   3. a muscle relaxant.
   4. an oxytocic.

3. Medications given to help stimulate milk to flow include
   1. oxytocics.
   2. muscle relaxants.
   3. tranquilizers.
   4. diuretics.

4. A medication used to expel the fetus from the pregnant uterus, used early in pregnancy, is called
   1. an abortifacient.
   2. a uterine relaxant.
   3. a muscle relaxant.
   4. an oxytocic.

WORKSHEET 20-3   Pituitary and Adrenocortical Hormones

1. Name two anterior pituitary hormones.

2. Name two posterior pituitary hormones.

3. The corticosteroids are composed of the _____ and the
    _____.

4. Identify five reasons one might want to give a corticosteroid.

    a.

    b.

    c.

    d.

    e.

5. List at least three routes for corticosteroid administration.

    a.

    b.

    c.

6. List at least five of the most common complications from long-term corticosteroid treatment.

7. What might happen if someone were to suddenly stop taking a corticosteroid after having taken it for a long time?

WORKSHEET 20-4   Sex Hormones

1. Androgens are used in weak and debilitated patients. Why?

2. Improvement in sexual development is (gradual, rapid).

3. Estrogens are used in what two common conditions?

4. The hormone given with estrogen in oral contraceptive pills is _____.

5. How do oral contraceptives work?

6. Adverse reactions to oral birth control pills are caused by _____.

7. List at least three symptoms of each.

    a. Estrogen excess

    b. Progestin excess

    c. Androgen excess

    d. Estrogen deficiency

    e. Progestin deficiency

(Continued)

WORKSHEET 20-4   Sex Hormones *(cont'd)*

8. List at least three contraindications to the use of oral birth control pills.

9. What is the difference between an absolute contraindication and a strong relative contraindication?

WORKSHEET 20-5   Thyroid Preparations

1. Ms. Larkin complains of weight gain, lack of appetite, and a dryness of her skin and hair. She also reports recent difficulty with constipation. The doctor suspects thyroid problems. Thyroid tests would probably show
    1. euthyroid.
    2. hyperthyroid.
    3. hypothyroid.
    4. normal thyroid.

2. An increase in thyroid hormone often produces weight loss in patients because
    1. patients lose their appetites and eat less.
    2. patients develop an inability to metabolize food.
    3. metabolic rate is increased.
    4. metabolic rate is decreased.

3. Define myxedema.
    1. A syndrome of doughy skin, puffy face, large tongue, and cool skin; may be associated with eye changes
    2. A syndrome of rapid pulse, irritability, decreased menses, nervousness, heat intolerance, and diarrhea
    3. A symptom where the eyes protrude and bulge
    4. A symptom where reflexes are increased

4. Patients with hypothyroidism are
    1. very sensitive to thyroid preparations.
    2. relatively intolerant of thyroid preparations.
    3. in need of iodine.

5. Antithyroid preparations are taken when
    1. the thyroid is enlarged and the doctor wants to help it return to its normal size.
    2. the synthesis of thyroid hormones must be stimulated.
    3. the patient has very slow reflexes and myxedema.
    4. synthesis of thyroid hormones must be inhibited.

6. Laboratory studies should be collected on patients with thyroid disease because the level of thyroid preparation in the blood
    1. must be monitored.
    2. must always be increased.
    3. must always be decreased.
    4. varies.

7. List at least three thyroid replacement hormones.

    a. _____

    b. _____

    c. _____

8. List two antithyroid drugs.

    a. _____

    b. _____

◆ Chapter 20—Integrated Case Study ◆

Lucy Bradford is a 33-year-old type 2 diabetic. She developed diabetes after a pregnancy 3 years ago, and she has been able to keep her blood glucose level under control with diet until recently. Her blood sugar has been around 136 mg/dL. Over the past few months, the glucose level has begun to vary a great deal, sometimes reaching as high as 180 mg/dL. She has no other health problems or previous surgeries but has smoked one pack of cigarettes a day for 12 years. She takes oral contraceptives. She reports developing a red itchy rash after taking sulfa as a child. Today the doctor decided she needed to start on some oral antidiabetic medication and ordered glyburide 5 mg/day PO.

1. What would you tell Lucy about the medication she is going to start taking?

2. Is this a low, medium, or high dose of glyburide?

3. What blood sugar level would be an appropriate goal for Lucy?

4. What blood test monitors the effectiveness of blood sugar control over a 6- to 8-week period?

5. From your knowledge of Lucy's condition and what you know about glyburide, how do you anticipate Lucy will react to the glyburide?

6. All sulfonylureas have the same mechanism of action. What differs is _____.

(Continued)

◆ Chapter 20—Integrated Case Study *(cont'd)* ◆

7. The physician decides to switch Lucy to _____ , which has a similar mechanism of action to the sulfonylureas. Why would this drug be a good substitute?

8. Lucy comes back several months later. Her glycohemoglobin A_{1c} is less than 7%. Is this a problem?

9. Diet and exercise are the foundation of any diabetes management plan. Develop a teaching plan for communicating these important things to Lucy:
   a. A more ideal body weight reduces insulin resistance and can significantly impact glucose control.
   b. The total number of calories that are adequate to promote a reasonable weight and good nutrition should be established.
   c. Generally, dividing the total number of calories into three smaller meals and 2 to 3 snacks minimizes postprandial glucose spikes. Spreading out calories may also control increased hunger associated with skipped meals.
   d. Generally 10% to 20% of the total daily calories are from protein, 20% of calories are from saturated and polyunsaturated fat, and 60% to 70% of calories are from monounsaturated fats and from carbohydrates.
   e. Exercise helps achieve and maintain an ideal body weight, resulting in decreased insulin resistance. Exercise also improves insulin sensitivity. For reasons not well understood, the exercising muscle requires little insulin but can mobilize moderate amounts of glucose.

10. Lucy's potential for hyperglycemia is increased because _____.

11. Lucy does not want to have another child. She has been taking a biphasic oral contraceptive pill. Are there any contraindications to diabetics taking oral contraceptive pills?

12. Does Lucy have any other risk factors that would limit oral contraceptive use?

Immunologic Medications

Answer Key: A complete answer key was provided for your instructor.

OBJECTIVES

1. Define common terms used in immunology.
2. Explain the differences between the three different types of immunity.
3. Outline typical immunization plans for children and adults.
4. List the major adverse reactions of common immunologic drugs.
5. Identify at least three drugs used for in vivo testing.

💿 **Be sure to check out the bonus material on the free CD-ROM in your textbook, including:**

Audio Pronunciation Guide
NCLEX®-Style Review Questions: Chapter 21
Top 200 Drugs by Prescription

WORKSHEET 21-1   Immunologic Agents

_____ results when a patient has an illness and then develops antibodies to the caus-ative agent.
1. Passive immunity
2. Naturally acquired active immunity
3. Antigen response
4. Artificially acquired active immunity

Bacteria that invade an individual may produce proteins called
1. vaccines.
2. toxins.
3. antitoxins.
4. venoms.

When a toxin or an antigen is weakened so that it may be given to an individual to provoke antibodies, we say it has been
1. artificially acquired.
2. naturally acquired.
3. attenuated.
4. strengthened.

When a vaccine is produced in the laboratory and given to individuals to help them develop immunity, the process is called
1. artificially acquired active immunity.
2. artificially acquired passive immunity.
3. naturally acquired active immunity.
4. naturally acquired passive immunity.

_____ is/are special collections of protein antibodies taken from blood serum or plas-ma and given to a person who does not have antibodies for a particular disease.
1. Albumin
2. Creatinine
3. Globulins
4. Alpha globulins

An example of a biologic product used in screening procedures to identify individuals exposed to a specific disease is
1. PPD.
2. rubeola.
3. tetanus toxoid.
4. hepatitis B.

The most common side effects of immunologic agents are
1. pain at the injection site and fever.
2. nausea, vomiting, GI distress, and diarrhea.
3. fever, hypertension, and seizures.
4. blood clots, anemia, and headaches.

(Continued)

WORKSHEET 21-1   Immunologic Agents *(cont'd)*

8. Because of the biologic source of some products, occasionally people may be unusually sensitive to immunologic products if they have allergy to
   1. eggs or feathers.
   2. grass pollen or trees.
   3. molds.
   4. aspirin or aspartame.

9. Sometimes immunity levels decrease over time. The result of this is that the patient
   1. remains immune to the organism.
   2. requires a booster immunization to raise immunity level.
   3. will eventually develop a mild case of the disease.
   4. will have life-long immunity as long as there is any antigen-antibody memory in the cells.

▶ Chapter 21—Integrated Case Study ◆

Mr. John Phillips, 53, a state highway patrol officer, discovered an injured raccoon along the highway. As he attempted to remove it from the road, the raccoon scratched and bit him. The raccoon was taken to the local animal control department, where it was discovered to be infected with rabies.

What treatment should Mr. Phillips receive?
1. Rabies vaccine
2. Rabies immune globulin
3. Need more information
4. Rabies vaccine and rabies immune globulin

Mr. Phillips tells you he has had prophylactic rabies injections. Does this make a difference in the treatment?
1. No. The treatment is the same.
2. Yes. In people who have had prophylaxis with rabies vaccine, give one dose of rabies vaccine but no rabies immune globulin.
3. Yes. In people who have had prophylaxis with rabies vaccine, give one dose of rabies vaccine and one dose of immune globulin.
4. Yes. In people who have had prophylaxis with rabies vaccine, give one dose of immune globulin.

What treatments may be required?
1. Immediate washing of the bite with soap and hot water
2. Cleaning the area vigorously with alcohol
3. Covering the bite area with sterile gauze
4. Injecting the antibiotic into the wound site

Administering rabies vaccine to Mr. Phillips is an example of what type of immunity?
1. Naturally acquired active immunity
2. Artificially acquired active immunity
3. Naturally acquired passive immunity
4. Artificially acquired passive immunity

Which groups of people would commonly be considered at high risk for rabies and thus should receive prophylactic therapy?
1. Truck drivers, police officers, firefighters
2. Veterinarians, animal handlers, certain laboratory workers
3. Food handlers
4. Health care workers

Antiinflammatory, Musculoskeletal, and Antiarthritis Medications

Answer Key: A complete answer key was provided for your instructor.

OBJECTIVES

1. List medications commonly used for the treatment of minor musculoskeletal pain and inflammation.
2. Identify the appropriate use for musculoskeletal relaxants.
3. Explain the mechanisms of action for different antiarthritis medications.
4. Describe the clinical situations in which uricosuric therapy may be indicated.
5. Compare the actions of various antiinflammatory and muscle relaxant agents.
6. Describe adverse reactions frequently found in the use of antiarthritis medications.

💿 **Be sure to check out the bonus material on the free CD-ROM in your textbook, including:**

Audio Pronunciation Guide
NCLEX®-Style Review Questions: Chapter 22
Top 200 Drugs by Prescription

WORKSHEET 22-1   Antiinflammatory Analgesic Agents

. Salicylates have _____, _____, and _____ effects.

. The medication with the greatest antiinflammatory effect of all salicylates is _____.

. Salicylates are most commonly used in the treatment of _____, _____, and _____.

. Less common uses are for treatment of _____ and _____.

. Two common adverse reactions to antiinflammatory analgesics include _____ and _____.

. Salicylates commonly interact with other medications to _____ effects of the other drugs.

. In ordering salicylates for a patient, the nurse would want to ask specifically about hypersensitivity to _____ and _____.

. Specimens for _____ may be required before the patient is started on salicylates because of the increased incidence of _____ in patients taking salicylates.

. Situations in which salicylate use might be contraindicated would include surgery, before labor, or in patients with transient ischemic attacks (TIAs) because _____.

0. Children with symptoms of recurrent upper respiratory infections, chickenpox, or influenza should not be given salicylates because of the positive association with development of _____.

1. Four-year-old Lisa Tilden is started on aspirin to control pain from a broken arm. You want to especially warn the parents that
   1. children under 12 are more prone to salicylate toxicity.
   2. she will need very large doses in order to control the pain.
   3. the aspirin will probably not help her pain.
   4. she should not force fluids while taking the medication.

2. In order to help avoid the development of salicylate toxicity in Lisa, you understand that
   1. small, frequent doses should be given.
   2. you should expect that Lisa will complain of ringing in her ears.
   3. adequate hydration is important in avoiding salicylate toxicity.
   4. she might develop Reye's syndrome.

3. Which of these patients can be given salicylates?
   1. Mr. Avarado, who has cirrhosis of the liver
   2. Mrs. Leido, who is in her second trimester of pregnancy
   3. Bobbie Feldman, who has the chicken pox

4. If a child swallows 3 or 4 aspirin tablets the parents should
   1. call poison control immediately.
   2. make the child vomit and then give him a glass of milk.
   3. take him to the hospital emergency room.
   4. the dosage is so low that it would not be a problem for a child.

(Continued)

WORKSHEET 22-1   Antiinflammatory Analgesic Agents *(cont'd)*

15. Angela Monsen broke her leg in a skiing accident. She has been taking medication for the pain for 2 weeks. You know that
    1. she is probably addicted to the medicine.
    2. the medicine ordered is not helping her.
    3. musculoskeletal pain that persists for more than 10 days automatically requires higher dosages of medication.
    4. this is not unusual.

16. In diabetic patients taking salicylates
    1. salicylates may give a false reading in those patients using Benedict's Clinitest.
    2. salicylates may give a false reading in those patients using a glucometer.
    3. salicylates have no effect on diabetic urine or blood tests.

17. Fred Scott is a mail carrier who takes salicylates for aching in his legs and feet. He is also a diabetic who has taken an oral hypoglycemic agent. You remember that
    1. salicylates cannot be taken with oral hypoglycemic agents.
    2. salicylates potentiate the action of oral hypoglycemic agents.
    3. salicylates weaken the action of oral hypoglycemic agents.
    4. oral hypoglycemic agents often increase the adverse effects of salicylates.

18. Tinnitus is described as a
    1. sharp pain in the ocular area.
    2. sensation of fullness in the ears.
    3. slight jerking movement of the eyes.
    4. ringing sensation in the ears.

19. The importance of tinnitus is that it is
    1. often the first sign of salicylate toxicity.
    2. present in almost every patient taking salicylates.
    3. useful in determining the appropriate dose of medicine.
    4. a sign that the patient is compliant with medication.

20. If tinnitus develops, the dosage should be _____ or _____.

21. How is dosage in arthritic patients determined?

22. Both salicylates and NSAIDs inhibit _____, which influences both _____ and _____.

23. Both salicylates and NSAIDs produce many adverse reactions in the _____.

24. Mr. Wixom has been taking NSAIDs for arthritis in his hands for several months. He feels there has been no relief of symptoms.
    1. You know that the dosage must be too low.
    2. If a patient fails to respond to a course of NSAIDs, it means there will be no improvement with a second NSAID agent.
    3. If a patient fails to respond to a course of NSAIDs, it means you may need to have a trial with a different NSAID.
    4. You know that he doesn't really have arthritis.

(Continued)

WORKSHEET 22-1   Antiinflammatory Analgesic Agents *(cont'd)*

5. The full therapeutic effect of an antiinflammatory agent may not be seen for
   1. 2 to 4 months.
   2. 1 to 2 weeks.
   3. 3 months.
   4. 6 weeks.

6. Richard Sutton has been taking NSAIDs regularly for a sports injury. He finds that the medications produce gastric irritation. You might tell him that
   1. taking the medications with food or milk helps to reduce the problems of gastric irritation.
   2. these medications should be taken on an empty stomach.
   3. gastric irritation cannot be avoided.
   4. his medication will need to be changed.

7. Clark Rockwood is a high school wrestler with a torn rotator cuff. He has a hard time remembering to take his medication because he is not feeling any pain. You tell him that
   1. he must take the medication or he will develop pain once he starts exercising.
   2. keeping a certain level of medicine within the blood at all times is important in maintaining the anti-inflammatory effect of the drugs.
   3. if he is not feeling any pain he does not need to take the medicine.
   4. he should only take the medication when he has pain with activity.

8. Clark should know that he might develop some side effects to the NSAID. You should tell him that
   1. blurred vision, ringing in the ears, or rashes should all be promptly reported to the physician.
   2. GI bleeding is the major problem to be concerned about.
   3. allergy to these medications is common for those who have a penicillin allergy.
   4. he must force fluids to avoid urate crystal precipitation in the kidney.

9. Mr. McComber, a retired baseball player, comes to the office complaining of long-term pain in his right elbow and shoulder. He has been taking ASA gr x or 650 mg bid for the last few months to relieve the pain. This has not been helpful. Your evaluation is that this patient
   1. has not been taking medication long enough for results to be seen.
   2. should be taking a higher dosage in order to relieve symptoms.
   3. should be switched to NSAIDs for long-term therapy.

WORKSHEET 22-2   Skeletal Muscle Relaxants

1. The main action of skeletal muscle relaxants is to
   1. decrease muscle tone and involuntary movement without loss of voluntary motor function.
   2. inhibit transmission of impulses in the motor pathway at the level of the effector muscle.
   3. increase the contractile mechanism of the skeletal muscle fibers (direct myotrophic action).

2. Skeletal muscle relaxants are used in all of the following situations except
   1. relieving pain in musculoskeletal disorders involving peripheral injury and inflammation.
   2. relieving pain in neurological disorders involving peripheral injury.
   3. reducing muscle tension in joints and ligaments.
   4. relief of pain in bursitis.

3. Common adverse reactions of skeletal muscle relaxants include all of the following except
   1. irritability and insomnia.
   2. abdominal pain, nausea, and GI distress.
   3. hypotension and syncope.
   4. flushing and tachycardia.

4. List some of the CNS depressants that are known to interact additively with skeletal muscle relaxants.

5. Long-term use of skeletal muscle relaxants is not recommended because _____.

True/False
6. T F Skeletal muscle relaxants come in both oral and parenteral form.
7. T F Injectable forms of skeletal muscle relaxants are purported to be more effective than oral medications.
8. T F Oral skeletal muscle relaxants are of questionable benefit in relieving symptoms.
9. T F Local tissue irritation may be caused by the oral form of the medications.

10. Occasionally an idiosyncratic reaction may follow the first dose of a skeletal muscle relaxant. Symptoms, seen within minutes or hours of the first dose, include
    1. severe nausea, vomiting, and weakness.
    2. temporary loss of vision, weakness, dizziness, and confusion.
    3. respiratory depression, confusion, and drowsiness.
    4. paradoxical excitation, insomnia, and tachycardia.

11. Skeletal muscle relaxants may cause all of the following except
    1. hepatotoxicity.
    2. nephrotoxicity.
    3. ototoxicity.
    4. blood dyscrasias.

(Continued

WORKSHEET 22-2   Skeletal Muscle Relaxants *(cont'd)*

12. If the skeletal muscle relaxant has been given for 45 days without any signs of improvement,
    1. discontinue the drug because it cannot be effective.
    2. increase the dosage to achieve better results.
    3. discontinue the drug due to an increased risk of hepatoxicity.
    4. switch to another skeletal muscle relaxant because the patient may have developed tolerance to the product.

True/False
13. T   F   Acuteness of the musculoskeletal disorder dictates the duration of drug use.
14. T   F   Gradually reduce the dosage of the drug before termination to avoid symptoms.
15. T   F   Abrupt termination of these drugs can cause withdrawal symptoms after long-term use.

WORKSHEET 22-3   Antiarthritis Medications

1. List at least three specific medications used in the treatment of severe rheumatoid arthritis.

2. What are the indications for use of these drugs?

3. How do these drugs work?

4. Why are these drugs reserved for the more progressive forms of arthritis?

5. Fill in the following chart indicating the adverse reactions most associated with each medication.

Medication	Adverse Reactions
Hydroxychloroquine sulfate	_____
Penicillamine	_____
Methotrexate	_____
Gold compounds	_____

6. One characteristic these four medications have in common is that the therapeutic effect may be seen

    _____.

7. Patients should be told that, if they take any of these drugs, there is a _____ of adverse reactions and they may _____ therapeutic effects.

(Continued)

WORKSHEET 22-3   Antiarthritis Medications *(cont'd)*

8. Given the adverse reactions of these medications, why would patients be willing to take them?

9. What is a nitritoid reaction?

10. What is appropriate intervention for nitritoid reaction?

WORKSHEET 22-4   Antigout Agents

1. What is a uricosuric agent?

2. What are the two mechanisms producing high uric acid levels in the body?

3. What other medication in addition to uricosurics is used in treating patients with acute high uric acid levels?

4. Probenecid has another action not related to gout. It acts to _____ _____.

5. A patient should not be started on uricosuric agents during an acute episode of gout. Why not?

True/False

6. T   F   Allopurinol inhibits the production of uric acid.
7. T   F   Colchicine is used when the diagnosis of gout through examination of joint fluid is not possible.
8. T   F   Colchicine has no direct effect on the serum uric acid level.
9. T   F   Salicylates should not be given concurrently with uricosuric drugs.
10. T   F   Podagra is a painful skin reaction caused by uricosuric agents.

◆ Chapter 22—Integrated Case Study ◆

Larry Stephenson is a 43-year-old Air Force colonel. He comes into the medical clinic complaining of severe back pain from a ruptured vertebral disc. The pain starts in his left buttock and travels down his left leg. He is sent home with the following medications:

Ibuprofen 800 mg q8h PO
Medrol Dose Pack as ordered for 7 days
Hydrocodone 5 mg q6h prn

1. Describe why each of these medications is ordered for this problem.

2. The dose of ibuprofen is very high. Why is this dose ordered? Mr. Stephenson returns to the clinic in 1 week. He is not feeling any better. He continues to have severe buttocks pain and has trouble sleeping. He also complains of severe itching.

3. The health care provider discontinues the hydrocodone and orders acetaminophen #2 with codeine. Why do you think she did this?

4. The health care provider also started the patient on orphenadrine (Norflex). Why was this medication ordered?

5. Does this patient have any contraindications to the use of this product?

(Continued)

◆ Chapter 22—Integrated Case Study *(cont'd)* ◆

6. Mr. Stephenson develops slight tachycardia, headache, dizziness, and blurred vision. Under questioning, he also reports increasing problems with constipation. Are these serious problems related to any of his medications?

7. Mr. Stephenson also reports that he has been having a lot of gastric burning. What is happening, and what can be done about it?

8. After a month, Mr. Stephenson still reports a little pain, particularly at night. He is feeling a little discouraged that he has not made a complete recovery. The health care provider starts him on amitriptyline. Why is this medication ordered?

Answer Key: A complete answer key was provided for your instructor.

OBJECTIVES

1. Identify major categories of medications used topically.
2. List at least three preparations used to treat eye, ear, and skin problems.
3. Describe specific administration techniques for topical products.

Be sure to check out the bonus material on the free CD-ROM in your textbook, including:

Audio Pronunciation Guide
NCLEX®-Style Review Questions: Chapter 23
Top 200 Drugs by Prescription

WORKSHEET 23-1   Topical Preparations

1. Billy Harris awoke this morning with a sore throat. He stayed home from school and rested in bed. His mother is most likely to give him
    1. a local topical anesthetic to reduce oral pain.
    2. an antiseptic mouthwash to kill germs.
    3. a cycloplegic to reduce pharyngeal pain.
    4. an antibiotic that Billy has left over from another illness.

2. When Melissa was born, the nurse put silver nitrate in her eyes. This is done to
    1. prevent bacterial infections from developing in Melissa's eyes.
    2. prevent gonorrheal ophthalmia neonatorum.
    3. avoid the possibility of *Chlamydia* infection in the baby.
    4. cleanse the baby's eyes from meconium.

3. Amanda Moore has been wearing contact lenses for 4 years. She has been studying late at night, and her eyes are very dry. The doctor may decide she needs to use
    1. a local anesthetic.
    2. antiseptic drops to reduce minor irritation.
    3. artificial tears.
    4. a topical antibiotic to reduce minor infection.

4. Name at least three types of medications used in treating glaucoma.

    a. _____

    b. _____

    c. _____

5. What is a precaution the nurse must consider in dilating a person's eyes?

6. How do antiglaucoma medications work to reduce problems of glaucoma?

7. Products used for the eye must be labeled
    1. otic preparation.
    2. otic or topical preparation.
    3. ophthalmic preparation.
    4. ophthalmic or otic preparation.

(Continued)

WORKSHEET 23-1   *Topical Preparations (cont'd)*

8. Richard Egan has noted reduced hearing for the last few months. The doctor tells him his ear is filled with wax. The doctor will probably order
   1. erythromycin.
   2. Debrox.
   3. hydrogen peroxide.
   4. Neo-Synephrine.

9. Match the following preparations with the topical disorder for which they might be used.

_____ Medicated bar soap	A.	Infected skin abrasion
_____ Burn preparations	B.	Minor cautery
_____ Zinc oxide stick	C.	Dandruff
_____ Sulfur preparation	D.	Scabies mite
_____ Emollients	E.	Treatment of psoriasis
_____ Topical antibiotic	F.	Contact dermatitis
_____ Keratolytic	G.	Dry skin
_____ Topical steroid	H.	Dry irritated skin
_____ Antipsoriatic	I.	Inflammatory skin condition
_____ Wet dressing	J.	Herpes simplex
_____ Antiseborrheic shampoo	K.	Second degree burn
_____ Acyclovir	L.	Acne
_____ Scabicides	M.	Head lice
_____ Pediculocides	N.	Seborrhea

10. Describe how to properly administer each of the following.

    Eyedrops

    Eye ointment

    Eardrops

◆ Chapter 23—Integrated Case Study ◆

Jenny Hawkes has worn contacts for over 30 years. She has ophthalmic examinations about every 2 years and has been relatively free of problems. When she had her last visit, the doctor told her she had a little conjunctivitis and ordered an antibiotic.

1.   What are some topical antiinfectives that might be ordered?

2.   On her yearly visits, the ophthalmologist measures the intraocular pressure and dilates her eyes to view the retina. This year, there is some evidence that Jenny is developing glaucoma. Is there any concern about dilating her eyes if she might be developing glaucoma?

3.   Why are there different categories of drugs used in the treatment of glaucoma?

4.   After several follow-up visits, Jenny is started on Timoptic. What kind of a medication is this, and what are some of the anticipated reactions to the drug?

5.   After a number of years taking Timoptic, the intraocular pressure again begins to rise. Is the disease process worsening? What is causing the change?

(Continued)

◆ Chapter 23—Integrated Case Study *(cont'd)* ◆

6. What other antiglaucoma products might Jenny take?

7. Do antiglaucoma products interfere with wearing contact lenses?

8. Jenny wakes up one morning with sharp, scratchy pains in her left eye. Her eye is tearing, and she is unable to keep it open. The eye doctor puts fluorescein sodium in her eye. Why?

9. The doctor discovers a small foreign body lodged in the cornea. It is removed with a needle, Jenny's eye is patched, and she is sent home. What types of medications might be required?

24 Vitamins and Minerals

Answer Key: A complete answer key was provided for your instructor.

OBJECTIVES

1. Identify the actions and indications for vitamins and minerals.
2. List at least six products used to treat vitamin or mineral deficiencies.
3. Present a teaching plan for patients who require vitamin or mineral supplements.

Be sure to check out the bonus material on the free CD-ROM in your textbook, including:

Audio Pronunciation Guide
NCLEX®-Style Review Questions: Chapter 24
Top 200 Drugs by Prescription

WORKSHEET 24-1   Vitamins

1. Vitamins are classified according to their solubility. Which vitamins are fat-soluble?

2. Although vitamins have been given a letter of the alphabet to identify them, they all have one or more scientific names, depending on the number of chemicals making up that vitamin category. Fill in the following chart with the proper names of the vitamins.

Vitamin	Other Names or Chemicals
Vitamin A	_____
Vitamin B_1	_____
Vitamin B_2	_____
Vitamin B_3	_____
Vitamin B_5	_____
Vitamin B_6	_____
Vitamin B_{12}	_____
Vitamin C	_____
Vitamin D	_____
Vitamin E	_____
Vitamin K	_____

3. What does DFI stand for?

True/False
4. T   F   The best vitamins are the most expensive vitamins.
5. T   F   Natural vitamins are better than synthetic vitamins.
6. T   F   A vitamin is a vitamin!

(Continued)

WORKSHEET 24-1 Vitamins *(cont'd)*

7. Name one major action or use of each of the following vitamins.

Vitamin	Major Action or Use
Vitamin A	_____
Vitamin B_1	_____
Vitamin B_2	_____
Vitamin B_3	_____
Vitamin B_5	_____
Vitamin B_6	_____
Vitamin B_{12}	_____
Vitamin C	_____
Vitamin D	_____
Vitamin E	_____
Vitamin K	_____

True/False

8. T F Vitamins come in different units: international units (IU), mg, or units (U).
9. T F Carrots are a good source of vitamin C.
10. T F Eating spinach is a good way to get lots of calcium.
11. T F Vitamin B_1 is easily leached out of food and destroyed by high heat.
12. T F Riboflavin and pyridoxine storage in the body is depleted by oral contraceptive pill use, so women taking the pill may need supplements.
13. T F Riboflavin deficiency is demonstrated by mucous-membrane, cutaneous, gastrointestinal, and CNS symptoms.
14. T F Good sources of pyridoxine include yeast, wheat, corn, egg yolk, liver, kidney, and muscle meats.
15. T F Irreparable neurologic damage may occur if B_{12} deficiency occurs longer than 3 months or when treatment for pernicious anemia includes only folic acid.

WORKSHEET 24-2   Minerals

1. The major difference between vitamins and minerals is that vitamins are (organic, inorganic) products and minerals are (organic, inorganic) products.

2. The Food and Nutrition Board of the National Research Council has established recommended daily intakes for _____ and _____.

3. The three minerals most often missing in the diet are _____ and _____ and _____.

4. Minerals essential in small quantities for metabolism include _____, _____, and _____.

5. _____ is a major mineral in the body essential for muscular and neurologic activity, repair of skeletal tissues, and activation of enzyme systems.

6. _____ is concentrated in bones and teeth and helps provide greater resistance to dissolution or demineralization.

7. An element important in the synthesis of myoglobin and hemoglobin is _____.

8. Trace elements _____ and _____ work in several enzyme systems.

9. Abnormalities of taste and smell, profound disinterest in food, delayed healing, and rough skin may be associated with _____ deficiency.

◆ Chapter 24—Integrated Case Study ◆

Mrs. Casper, age 77, has been in a nursing home for several years. She suffers from a variety of chronic diseases. When she was recently admitted to the hospital for pneumonia, the physician discovered that she was mildly anemic. She was prescribed the following:

Ferrous sulfate: 300 mg 3 times daily PO
Vitamin C: 1000 mcg daily
Ciprofloxacin: 750 mg PO q12h

1. Why is the ferrous sulfate ordered?

2. Why is vitamin C given?

3. Why is ciprofloxacin given?

4. After several days of therapy, the patient does not seem to be getting any better. Can you determine any reason why this might be so?

5. The patient is switched to another antibiotic and eventually goes home to stay with her son and grandchildren. Her 4-year-old granddaughter opens her ferrous sulfate and swallows 8 tablets. What should be done? Why?

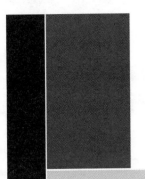

FDA Categories for Drug Use in Pregnancy

Category	Description
A	Adequate, well-controlled studies in pregnant women have not shown an increased risk of fetal abnormalities.
B	Animal studies have revealed no evidence of harm to the fetus; however, there are no adequate and well-controlled studies in pregnant women. **OR** Animal studies have shown an adverse effect, but adequate and well-controlled studies in pregnant women have failed to demonstrate a risk to the fetus.
C	Animal studies have shown an adverse effect and there are no adequate and well-controlled studies in pregnant women. **OR** No animal studies have been conducted and there are no adequate and well-controlled studies in pregnant women.
D	Studies, adequate well-controlled or observational, in pregnant women have demonstrated a risk to the fetus. However, the benefits of therapy may outweigh the potential risk.
X	Studies, adequate well-controlled or observational, in animals or pregnant women have demonstrated positive evidence of fetal abnormalities. The use of the product is contraindicated in women who are or may become pregnant.

From Meadows M: Pregnancy and the drug dilemma, *FDA Consumer magazine*, 2001. Available at www.fda.gov/fdac/features/2001/301 preg.html#categories, accessed June 2005.

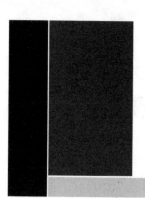

The Top 200 Prescriptions by Number of US Prescriptions Dispensed

Drug Name	Total Prescriptions	Drug Name	Total Prescriptions
HYDROCODONE W/APAP	92,719,975	LEVOXYL	19,760,520
LIPITOR	69,766,431	LORAZEPAM	18,873,635
LISINOPRIL	46,206,563	ALLEGRA	18,772,070
ATENOLOL	44,162,229	PLAVIX	18,721,885
SYNTHROID	44,056,176	EFFEXOR XR	18,574,507
AMOXICILLIN	41,393,538	POTASSIUM CHLORIDE	18,523,548
HYDROCHLOROTHIAZIDE	41,345,733	PROTONIX	18,359,740
ZITHROMAX	37,171,754	PROPOXYPHENE NAP W/APAP	17,931,369
FUROSEMIDE	36,508,251	ADVAIR DISKUS	17,400,826
NORVASC	34,729,004	WARFARIN SODIUM	16,581,657
TOPROL XL	32,794,562	ACETAMINOPHEN W/ CODEINE	16,079,867
ALPRAZOLAM	32,404,743	CLONAZEPAM	15,968,529
ALBUTEROL	31,219,862	NEURONTIN	15,476,692
ZOLOFT	29,877,707	FLONASE	15,136,691
ZOCOR	27,234,005	AMITRIPTYLINE HCL	15,086,803
METFORMIN HCL	25,472,580	RANITIDINE HCL	14,884,810
IBUPROFEN	25,188,051	TRAZODONE HCL	14,450,339
TRIAMTERENE W/HCTZ	24,616,014	NAPROXEN (FDA alert issued December 2004)	13,918,496
AMBIEN	24,494,669	AMOX TR-POTASSIUM CLAVULANATE	13,810,927
CEPHALEXIN	23,665,172	ENALAPRIL MALEATE	13,732,556
NEXIUM	23,641,811	PAROXETINE HCL	13,731,071
PREVACID	23,628,587	PRAVACHOL	13,662,403
LEXAPRO	22,597,383	VIAGRA	13,539,272
PREDNISONE	22,506,888	CYCLOBENZAPRINE HCL	13,246,157
ZYRTEC	22,382,823	VIOXX (Recalled October 2004)	13,226,546
SINGULAIR	22,020,478	ALTACE	13,149,598
CELEBREX (FDA advisory issued December 2004)	21,916,220	DIOVAN	13,133,513
FLUOXETINE HCL	21,752,487	LOTREL	13,037,546
FOSAMAX	20,972,548	LEVAQUIN	12,926,850
METOPROLOL TARTRATE	20,840,044		
PREMARIN	20,324,619		

Drug Name	Total Prescriptions	Drug Name	Total Prescriptions
L-THYROXINE SODIUM	12,394,756	COUMADIN	7,707,865
BEXTRA (*Recalled April 2005*)	12,227,513	ADDERALL XR	7,707,093
OXYCODONE W/APAP	12,118,687	CONCERTA	7,618,920
DIAZEPAM	12,093,060	NASONEX	7,605,041
TRAMADOL HCL	11,852,004	CLARINEX	7,577,701
VERAPAMIL HCL	11,143,691	LOVASTATIN	7,373,795
DIOVAN HCT	10,737,750	HYZAAR	7,340,635
ALBUTEROL SULFATE	10,498,863	SPIRONOLACTONE	7,271,450
LISINOPRIL/HCTZ	10,406,078	AMARYL	7,246,808
ORTHO EVRA	10,380,213	DIGITEK	7,225,219
CELEXA	10,358,042	TEMAZEPAM	7,134,429
ACCUPRIL	10,236,306	DIFLUCAN	7,107,234
CARISOPRODOL	9,947,523	EVISTA	7,085,682
ACTOS	9,875,273	XALATAN	7,075,287
PROMETHAZINE HCL	9,725,896	LANTUS	7,009,424
ACTONEL	9,723,277	COREG	6,961,217
ISOSORBIDE MONONITRATE	9,621,678	COMBIVENT	6,888,620
ALLOPURINOL	9,537,507	CRESTOR	6,887,980
PAXIL CR	9,507,161	COTRIM	6,800,424
COZAAR	9,501,756	VALTREX	6,782,224
CLONIDINE HCL	9,451,698	ZYPREXA	6,498,677
CIPROFLOXACIN HCL	9,366,605	DOXAZOSIN MESYLATE	6,485,905
WELLBUTRIN XL	9,260,409	OXYCONTIN	6,386,235
GLYBURIDE	9,227,291	TRIAMCINOLONE ACETONIDE	6,378,669
AVANDIA	9,194,550	ESTRADIOL	6,356,120
PENICILLIN VK	9,044,304	ASPIRIN	6,280,399
ZETIA	8,969,666	ALLEGRA-D 12 HOUR	6,267,316
TRIMOX	8,904,667	ENDOCET	6,247,225
METHYLPREDNISOLONE	8,695,743	GEMFIBROZIL	6,161,194
FOLIC ACID	8,640,505	ORTHO TRI-CYCLEN	6,028,942
ACIPHEX	8,531,810	METOCLOPRAMIDE HCL	6,024,790
GLIPIZIDE ER	8,526,225	HYDROXYZINE HCL	5,976,840
FLOMAX	8,502,798	AVAPRO	5,905,598
DILTIAZEM HCL	8,501,749	ORTHO TRI-CYCLEN LO	5,825,865
RISPERDAL	8,458,338	TOPAMAX	5,799,851
OMEPRAZOLE	8,449,378	IMITREX	5,764,066
YASMIN 28	8,328,815	STRATTERA	5,762,842
DOXYCYCLINE HYCLATE	8,225,902	METFORMIN HCL ER	5,749,616
TRICOR	8,058,816	DETROL LA	5,740,205
SEROQUEL	7,952,278	OMNICEF	5,640,331

Drug Name	Total Prescriptions	Drug Name	Total Prescriptions
MECLIZINE HCL	5,621,298	MOBIC	4,441,328
TRINESSA	5,607,134	DURAGESIC	4,409,435
FLOVENT	5,605,531	ACYCLOVIR	4,333,297
GLIPIZIDE	5,579,469	FAMOTIDINE	4,287,821
PROPOXYPHENE NAPSYLATE W/APAP	5,563,827	HUMULIN N	4,261,396
ULTRACET	5,558,854	NIASPAN	4,246,644
CLINDAMYCIN HCL	5,536,403	DIGOXIN	4,217,773
METRONIDAZOLE	5,415,244	FERROUS SULFATE	4,197,333
LANOXIN	5,264,880	NECON	4,150,286
NYSTATIN	5,111,085	AVIANE	4,113,691
BISOPROLOL FUMARATE/ HCTZ	5,047,342	DICLOFENAC SODIUM	4,072,977
DEPAKOTE	5,001,556	HUMALOG	4,048,108
KLOR-CON	4,936,081	ELIDEL (*FDA advisory issued March 2005*)	4,018,917
SMZ-TMP	4,840,584	FLUCONAZOLE	4,012,259
BENAZEPRIL HCL	4,834,783	LORATADINE	4,003,152
MINOCYCLINE HCL	4,768,055	PATANOL	3,958,967
NASACORT AQ	4,750,255	BENICAR	3,918,409
CARTIA XT	4,745,853	CLOTRIMAZOLE/ BETAMETHASONE	3,886,738
MIRTAZAPINE	4,695,186	KLOR-CON M20	3,867,439
WELLBUTRIN SR	4,680,879	BIAXIN XL	3,821,600
RHINOCORT AQUA	4,633,208	TRI-SPRINTEC	3,783,480
PROPRANOLOL HCL	4,628,997	METHOTREXATE	3,753,232
PROMETHAZINE W/CODEINE	4,628,888	LAMICTAL	3,734,346
TERAZOSIN HCL	4,578,163	QUININE SULFATE	3,696,998
BUPROPION HCL	4,557,355	DILANTIN	3,624,606
PREMPRO	4,517,080	FOSINOPRIL SODIUM	3,582,773
ARICEPT	4,504,355	AMOXIL	3,567,624
LEVOTHROID	4,504,208	MIRALAX	3,565,964
BUSPIRONE HCL	4,488,014	PULMICORT	3,542,264
SKELAXIN	4,441,925	KETOCONAZOLE	3,541,303

For 2004. Based upon more than 3 billion prescriptions: Data furnished by NDC Health

Modified from *The Top 300 Prescriptions for 2004 by Number of US Prescriptions Dispensed*, Copyright © 2005 by RxList Inc.

Medication Cards

These sample medication cards have been printed on the front and back of this page so they can be easily repro-duced for student use. We recommend they be photocopied double-sided and cut into 4" by 6" cards.

Drug Name: _____ Trade Name: _____
Major Drug Category: _____
Drug Action: _____
_____
Uses: _____
_____
Adverse Reactions: _____
_____
Drug Interactions: _____
_____
Usual Drug Dosage: _____

Nursing Implications:
Assessment: _____
Diagnosis: _____
Planning: _____
Implementation: _____
Evaluation: _____

Drug Name: _____ Trade Name: _____
Major Drug Category: _____
Drug Action: _____
_____
Uses: _____
_____
Adverse Reactions: _____
_____
Drug Interactions: _____
_____
Usual Drug Dosage: _____

Nursing Implications:
Assessment: _____
Diagnosis: _____
Planning: _____
Implementation: _____
Evaluation: _____

Patient ID   Diagnosis   Comments Re: Administration/Patient Response

_____

_____

_____

_____

_____

_____

_____

_____

_____

_____

_____

_____

_____

_____

_____

Patient ID   Diagnosis   Comments Re: Administration/Patient Response

_____

_____

_____

_____

_____

_____

_____

_____

_____

_____

_____

_____

_____

_____

_____

Drug Name: _____ Trade Name: _____
Major Drug Category: _____
Drug Action: _____
_____
Uses: _____
_____
Adverse Reactions: _____
_____
Drug Interactions: _____
_____
Usual Drug Dosage: _____

Nursing Implications:
Assessment: _____
Diagnosis: _____
Planning: _____
Implementation: _____
Evaluation: _____

Drug Name: _____ Trade Name: _____
Major Drug Category: _____
Drug Action: _____
_____
Uses: _____
_____
Adverse Reactions: _____
_____
Drug Interactions: _____
_____
Usual Drug Dosage: _____

Nursing Implications:
Assessment: _____
Diagnosis: _____
Planning: _____
Implementation: _____
Evaluation: _____

Patient ID   Diagnosis   Comments Re: Administration/Patient Response

Patient ID   Diagnosis   Comments Re: Administration/Patient Response

Drug Name: _____ Trade Name: _____

Major Drug Category: _____

Drug Action: _____

_____

Uses: _____

_____

Adverse Reactions: _____

_____

Drug Interactions: _____

_____

Usual Drug Dosage: _____

Nursing Implications:

Assessment: _____

Diagnosis: _____

Planning: _____

Implementation: _____

Evaluation: _____

Drug Name: _____ Trade Name: _____

Major Drug Category: _____

Drug Action: _____

_____

Uses: _____

_____

Adverse Reactions: _____

_____

Drug Interactions: _____

_____

Usual Drug Dosage: _____

Nursing Implications:

Assessment: _____

Diagnosis: _____

Planning: _____

Implementation: _____

Evaluation: _____

Patient ID	Diagnosis	Comments Re: Administration/Patient Response

Patient ID	Diagnosis	Comments Re: Administration/Patient Response

Drug Name: _____ Trade Name: _____

Major Drug Category: _____

Drug Action: _____

_____

Uses: _____

_____

Adverse Reactions: _____

_____

Drug Interactions: _____

_____

Usual Drug Dosage: _____

Nursing Implications:

Assessment: _____

Diagnosis: _____

Planning: _____

Implementation: _____

Evaluation: _____

Drug Name: _____ Trade Name: _____

Major Drug Category: _____

Drug Action: _____

_____

Uses: _____

_____

Adverse Reactions: _____

_____

Drug Interactions: _____

_____

Usual Drug Dosage: _____

Nursing Implications:

Assessment: _____

Diagnosis: _____

Planning: _____

Implementation: _____

Evaluation: _____

Patient ID	Diagnosis	Comments Re: Administration/Patient Response

Patient ID	Diagnosis	Comments Re: Administration/Patient Response

Drug Name: _____ Trade Name: _____

Major Drug Category: _____

Drug Action: _____

_____

Uses: _____

_____

Adverse Reactions: _____

_____

Drug Interactions: _____

_____

Usual Drug Dosage: _____

Nursing Implications:

Assessment: _____

Diagnosis: _____

Planning: _____

Implementation: _____

Evaluation: _____

Drug Name: _____ Trade Name: _____

Major Drug Category: _____

Drug Action: _____

_____

Uses: _____

_____

Adverse Reactions: _____

_____

Drug Interactions: _____

_____

Usual Drug Dosage: _____

Nursing Implications:

Assessment: _____

Diagnosis: _____

Planning: _____

Implementation: _____

Evaluation: _____

Patient ID	Diagnosis	Comments Re: Administration/Patient Response

Patient ID	Diagnosis	Comments Re: Administration/Patient Response

Drug Name: _____ Trade Name: _____

Major Drug Category: _____

Drug Action: _____

_____

Uses: _____

_____

Adverse Reactions: _____

_____

Drug Interactions: _____

_____

Usual Drug Dosage: _____

Nursing Implications:

Assessment: _____

Diagnosis: _____

Planning: _____

Implementation: _____

Evaluation: _____

Drug Name: _____ Trade Name: _____

Major Drug Category: _____

Drug Action: _____

_____

Uses: _____

_____

Adverse Reactions: _____

_____

Drug Interactions: _____

_____

Usual Drug Dosage: _____

Nursing Implications:

Assessment: _____

Diagnosis: _____

Planning: _____

Implementation: _____

Evaluation: _____

Patient ID   Diagnosis   Comments Re: Administration/Patient Response
_____
_____
_____
_____
_____
_____
_____
_____
_____
_____
_____
_____
_____
_____
_____
_____
_____

Patient ID   Diagnosis   Comments Re: Administration/Patient Response
_____
_____
_____
_____
_____
_____
_____
_____
_____
_____
_____
_____
_____
_____
_____
_____
_____

Drug Name: _____ Trade Name: _____

Major Drug Category: _____

Drug Action: _____

_____

Uses: _____

_____

Adverse Reactions: _____

_____

Drug Interactions: _____

_____

Usual Drug Dosage: _____

Nursing Implications:

Assessment: _____

Diagnosis: _____

Planning: _____

Implementation: _____

Evaluation: _____

Drug Name: _____ Trade Name: _____

Major Drug Category: _____

Drug Action: _____

_____

Uses: _____

_____

Adverse Reactions: _____

_____

Drug Interactions: _____

_____

Usual Drug Dosage: _____

Nursing Implications:

Assessment: _____

Diagnosis: _____

Planning: _____

Implementation: _____

Evaluation: _____

Patient ID   Diagnosis   Comments Re: Administration/Patient Response

_____

_____

_____

_____

_____

_____

_____

_____

_____

_____

_____

_____

_____

_____

_____

_____

Patient ID   Diagnosis   Comments Re: Administration/Patient Response

_____

_____

_____

_____

_____

_____

_____

_____

_____

_____

_____

_____

_____

_____

_____

_____